Healthy Schools Healthy Futures

The Case for Improving School Environment

Alan C. Henderson, DrPH, CHES

ETR ASSOCIATES
Santa Cruz, California
1993

ETR Associates (Education, Training and Research) is a nonprofit organization committed to fostering the health, well-being and cultural diversity of individuals, families, schools and communities. The publishing program of ETR Associates provides books and materials that empower young people and adults with the skills to make positive health choices. We invite health professionals to learn more about our high-quality publishing, training and research programs by contacting us at P.O. Box 1830, Santa Cruz, CA 95061-1830.

About the Author

Alan C. Henderson, DrPH, CHES, is professor of health science at California State University, Long Beach. He has been involved in professional preparation of health educators for many years. He served as director of the Role Delineation Project for Health Education at the National Center for Health Education. He has worked with numerous professional and community organizations to improve preparation of health educators and meet the health education needs of the public.

© 1993 by ETR Associates. All rights reserved.

Published by ETR Associates, P.O. Box 1830, Santa Cruz, California 95061-1830

Printed in the United States of America
10 9 8 7 6 5 4 3 2 1

Cover design by Detta Penna
Text design by Ann Smiley

Title No. 598

Library of Congress Cataloging-in-Publication Data
Henderson, Alan C.
    Healthy schools, healthy futures : the case for improving school environment / Alan C. Henderson.
      p. cm.
    1. School hygiene—United States. 2. School children—Health and hygiene—United States. 3. Health education—United States. 4. School environment—United States. I. Title.
LB3409.U5H46 1993   92-36117
371.7'0973—dc20

Contents

Acknowledgments vii
Introduction 1

Chapter 1. The Importance of Healthy School Environments ... 3
    Health is Vital 4
    The Schools' Responsibility for Health and Safety 8
    School Environments at Risk 10

Chapter 2. How Healthy Are Our Schools? 13
    How Healthy Are Our Students? 14
    How Healthy Are School Personnel? 19
    Rising Health Care Costs 23
    Health Promotion for Staff—A Key to a Healthy
        Environment 24

Chapter 3. The Total Environment Concept 27
    The Culture of the School 28
    What Does the Environment Communicate? 30
    The Social Environment—A Crucial Component 31
    The Importance of Models 35
    Messages That Support Health 37
    Commitment—A Key Ingredient 38

Chapter 4. Partnerships for Change 41
    Key Roles at the School 44
    Building Partnerships for Change 50

Chapter 5. Schoolsite Health Promotion 55
    Why Schoolsite Health Promotion Programs? 56
    Key Ingredients for Successful Programs 57
    Benefits of Schoolsite Health Promotion Programs 64

Chapter 6. Taking Action to Improve the School Environment 67
    Forming a School Health Council 68
    Planning 72
    Implementation 76
    Evaluation 82
    Responding to Change 84
    Strategic Planning 87
    Special Considerations 88

Chapter 7. Success Stories: Making Things Work 91
    Coping with Changes in Family Structures and
        Student Populations...92
    Preventing and Controlling Violence 96
    Improving School Safety 100
    Retaining Students 102
    Improving Teacher Retention and Morale 103
    Working with Community Groups..105

Appendix A. Options for Change 109
Appendix B. Health Promotion Program Development 113
Appendix C. Strategic Plan Outline 117
Appendix D. Resources 123
Bibliography 127

Figures

Important Definitions 6
Elementary and Secondary School Personnel 20
Health Status of School Personnel 21
How Is Your School's Social Climate? 32
The Eight Components of Comprehensive School Health Programs 42
Content Areas for Comprehensive Health Education 43
Partnership Resources 54
Health Promotion Program Development 62
Action Steps Timeline 64
Benefits of Health Promotion 65
Creating a Foundation for Change 72
Sample Goals for a School Health Program 75
Suggested Initial Activities 79
Physical Hazards in the Schools 80

Acknowledgments

This book is the byproduct of numerous interactions with many colleagues in health education, education and health services over a long period of time. The genesis of this book can be traced to Ned Johns, who opened up the field of health education for me and reinforced my observations of and interactions with leaders in health education. It was precipitated by the interest, involvement and encouragement of my editors, Kathleen Middleton, Netha Thacker and Suzanne Schrag, and made possible by allowances of my family. Without my family's and editors' patience and encouragement during a particularly stressful period, this book would not have happened.

Additionally, I would like to acknowledge Sally Champlin, Nathan Matza and Mike Smith, who helped with the last chapter, and the professionals who reviewed manuscript and collaborated in a variety of ways:

David A. Birch, PhD
Director of Health Outreach
   Programs
Pennsylvania State University

Ric Loya
Teacher
Huntington Park High School
Huntington Park, California

Sherman K. Sowby, PhD
Professor of Health Science
California State University, Fresno

Robert Wanberg, PhD
State Director of Health Education
Minnesota Department of
   Education

Introduction

WE LIVE IN A remarkably turbulent environment. Social, economic and political structures have been altered and the demographic characteristics of our country have been broadened by an increasingly aging population and increases in ethnic and cultural diversity in groups and numbers. All of these rapid social changes have produced unprecedented pressures on our system of education, both private and public. School board members, superintendents, principals, teachers, staff and students confront demands to change the schools to meet a myriad of differing and often conflicting agendas.

This book addresses the school as a worksite for faculty, staff and administrators, as a learning site for students, and as an important site for creating a healthy, productive environment. Millions of students and school personnel spend a considerable amount of the day at school. The physical condition of the school, its psychological and social climate, and its efforts to protect, promote and improve health become important components of the daily lives of students and staff. Environmental factors have the potential to make real contributions to successful teaching/learning outcomes, as well as to preserve the health of the most essential resources for education—students, teachers, staff and administrators.

This book was born out of years of interest in and commitment to health education as an essential strategy for maintaining public health. Schools are vital resources for public health; ideally, students will graduate into adult roles as productive members of society. Years of education completed is directly linked to health status. That is, a greater number of years of education completed yields healthier individuals.

Our society faces the challenge of retaining quality of life for an ever-expanding population. Schools are one of the most important foundations for realizing this ambitious goal. A safe and healthy school environment is an essential ingredient in making it possible for schools to fulfill their roles as contributors to the nation's health.

This book is intended for all who have an interest in schools. Teachers, administrators, school board members, parents, representatives of community groups, and state, county and local educational agency representatives can use this book as a guide for conceptualizing and initiating school improvement. College and university faculty with responsibilities for preservice education of teachers, health educators and other school personnel may find the contents of the book useful for illustrating and expanding the concept of the school beyond teaching/learning transactions.

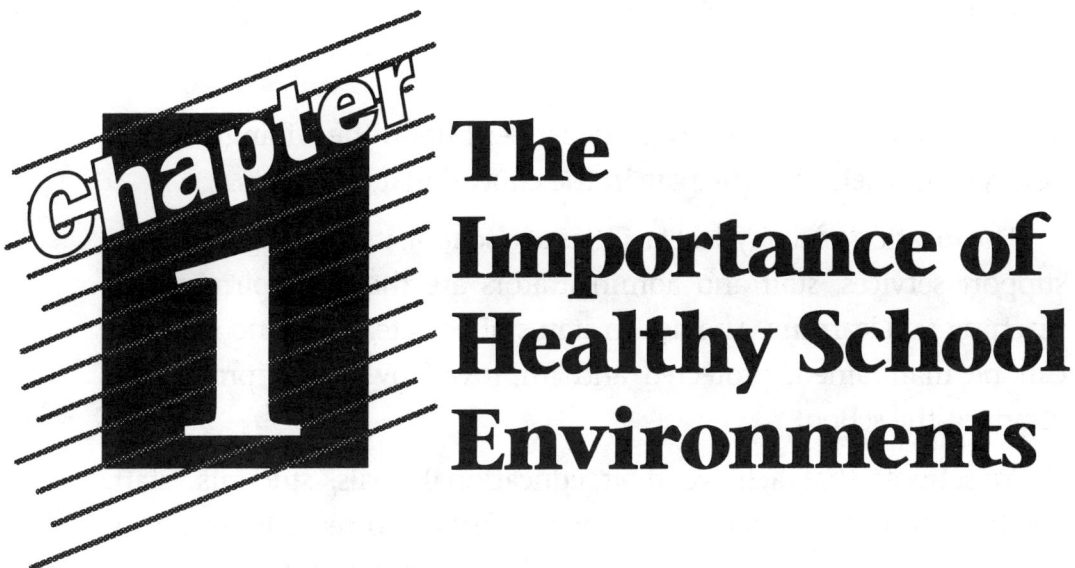

Chapter 1: The Importance of Healthy School Environments

AMERICAN SCHOOLS ARE COMPLEX organizations that offer their students a variety of different experiences. But they share a unified purpose in helping to socialize children and youth into responsible adult roles. The physical, emotional and social environments of a school have important effects on what students learn.

Much attention is paid to the teaching/learning process in schools. Its assessment and improvement dominate discussion. Educational reform and restructuring proposals have occupied the nation's attention in the 1980s and the early years of the 1990s. These proposals are aimed at helping schools to better prepare children and youth for responsible adulthood in American society. But very few of these proposals have looked upon the school as the important worksite that it is, or recognized that the school environment is a major element in educational success.

Education is a labor-intensive endeavor. Millions of students, teachers, administrators and staff spend their working days at schools throughout the United States. The quality of the teaching/learning process is determined by the skills and knowledge of those responsible

Healthy Schools, Healthy Futures

The Importance of Healthy School Environments

for education. The outcomes are dependent upon the willingness and ability of learners to participate in the educational process.

The location and physical facilities of a school, its learning resources, support services, staff and administrators are the underpinnings of teaching and learning. The health status of both teachers and students can be maintained, protected and improved by health promotion efforts at the school.

In schools that achieve their educational goals, students, staff, parents and outside groups work as a coordinated team in an atmosphere of mutual support and respect. In these schools, the teaching/learning process is a dynamic experience for students and teachers. All involved share feelings of enthusiasm and dedication.

These schools have resources that represent state-of-the-art technology to complement the school's programs. The physical plant is well cared for and has been adapted to meet the changing needs of the current population of students and staff. Graduates of the school are successfully placed in other educational or work environments. Staff have long, stable careers with high levels of job satisfaction, low turnover, high levels of productivity, and a robust outlook on education.

Does this environment really exist? Yes, it does, in schools in a variety of areas, including inner cities. Furthermore, these schools have used existing resources to create such environments. They have not depended on substantial outside fiscal, human and material support. How do such schools create an ideal setting for students and staff?

Health Is Vital

The foundation for improving the environment of the school is the recognition that the health of all those learning and working at school is vital to the educational process. Health was identified as one of the seven cardinal principles of education more than a hundred years ago. It is instrumental to all of our activities. Without a basic level of health, it's impossible to do all we need and want to do.

Most of us are familiar with the particular health concerns affecting children and youth, including the following:

- communicable and noncommunicable disease
- intended and unintended injury
- hearing, vision and ambulatory limitations
- early sexual behavior and pregnancy
- sexually transmitted disease, including HIV and AIDS
- alcohol and other drug dependencies
- behavioral problems

Each of these concerns is well described in popular and scientific media. However, concepts that can help educators link these issues and concerns together have been missing.

Over the last several years, an evolution of thought has begun to crystallize and shape approaches to these numerous health concerns. For example, a few years ago a California legislator formed a statewide commission on self-esteem. While there was much discussion in the popular press about the merits of this effort, the concept of self-esteem was seen as a common thread for many of the problems of California youth. Thus, the concept could be used to attack many concerns on a broad basis.

Similarly, the field of health education has embarked on an effort to develop standardized terminology for use in any health education setting (e.g., schools, public health departments, voluntary health agencies). This terminology should help those working in different settings coordinate their efforts. These definitions of health emphasize health as integral to other aspects of life. They focus on the interdependence of the physical, mental and social dimensions of health.

Important Definitions

Health
- A state of complete physical, mental and social well-being, and not merely the absence of disease and infirmity.
- A quality of life involving dynamic interaction and independence among the individual's physical well-being, his [sic] mental and emotional reactions, and the social complex in which he [sic] exists.
- An integrated method of functioning which is oriented toward maximizing the potential of which the individual is capable. It requires that the individual maintain a continuum of balance and purposeful direction with the environment where he [sic] is functioning.
- A set of health-enhancing behaviors, shaped by internally consistent values, attitudes, beliefs and external social and cultural forces.

Health Promotion and Disease Prevention
- The aggregate of all purposeful activities designed to improve personal and public health through a combination of strategies, including the competent implementation of behavioral change strategies, health education, health protection measures, risk factor detection, health enhancement and health maintenance.

Healthy Lifestyle
- A set of health-enhancing behaviors, shaped by internally consistent values, attitudes, beliefs and external social and cultural forces.

Comprehensive School Health Program
- An organized set of policies, procedures and activities designed to protect and promote the health and well-being of students and staff which has traditionally included health services, healthful school environment [emphasis added] and health education. It should also include, but not be limited to, guidance and counseling, physical education, food service, social work, psychological services and employee health promotion.

From the Report of the 1990 Joint Committee on Health Education Terminology. *Journal of Health Education* 22 (2): 97–108.

Such concepts of health make it possible to understand how disease processes are linked to individuals' characteristics and their behavior in social and emotional contexts. For example, alcohol and other drug dependencies are a product of the interaction of a drug, the physical and emotional aspects of the individual who is using the drug, and the social context in which the drug is made available and used.

The definition of a healthy lifestyle underscores these definitions of health and the ways health is manifested in practice. The definition connects internal processes with social and cultural influences. Understanding the factors that shape health practices helps us see how health behaviors may be introduced, reinforced and modified in the physical, emotional and social environment of our schools.

Health promotion and disease prevention assist the development of healthy lifestyles. Health promotion and disease prevention, as defined, include basic measures such as the following:

- screening for health problems and risk factors (e.g., vision, hearing, blood pressure, serum cholesterol)
- health protection through immunizations
- behavior changes such as diet, weight control and smoking cessation
- health maintenance and enhancement through self-care and habitual exercise.

The school site is an excellent locale for these activities. Such programs help meet the important goals of health promotion and disease prevention. Comprehensive school health programs attempt to join traditional school health services (nursing and food service), health instruction (substance use and abuse) and the school environment (school facilities, emotional and social climate) into an interrelated whole.

Health for all in our schools is inseparable from educational processes. Students cannot properly learn if they have health difficulties. Similarly, teachers and other school personnel cannot be effective if

The Importance of Healthy School Environments

they, too, face obstacles to health. Our broadened understanding of successful teaching/learning strategies for health recognizes the need for life-skills development. Such development enables students to analyze their social and physical environments. Students need to learn how to make healthy choices in environments that sometimes offer many unhealthy options.

The School's Responsibility for Health and Safety

Schools' basic responsibilities include protecting and promoting the health and safety of all who attend, not only students, but teachers, administrators and other staff as well. A school is made up of not only the physical plant and grounds, but also facilities, equipment, books, curricular materials, consumable supplies and people. Responsibilities for health and safety begin when new schools are planned and continue until a school is no longer used for education.

In legal terms, schools occupy a unique niche among society's organizations. School officials have the legal and ethical responsibility for looking after the health and safety of the young people who are their students. The schools act *in loco parentis,* meaning the schools take the place of the parents in a special way.

Schools are obligated to return students to parents or guardians at the end of the school day with the same health status students had when they left home to go to school. Schools are responsible for children and youth on the way to and from school, as well as during the school day. This responsibility requires that teachers and administrators take positive action in two ways.

First, school personnel must take reasonable steps to protect students from hazards that could be created by the physical environment of the school building and its surroundings. They must also protect students from hazards created by their own actions or those of others. Children and youth frequently act impulsively or fail to think through the risks they may encounter. Because school personnel should understand these qualities of young people, they are accountable for dealing with and removing harmful situations, whether physical, personal or interpersonal. Second, the school must establish discipline policies that hold students accountable for their actions.

Both aspects of the school's responsibility to its students require that teachers and administrators, as well as any other designated school officials, supervise the conduct of students and exert control to avert harm. Therefore, schools need to provide active supervision and enough supervising school personnel to reduce or eliminate risks as much as possible.

The importance of this ethical and legal obligation of school personnel warrants annual review, discussion and revision of school policies and procedures to identify the best means for protecting students. Administrators and teachers new to the school, as well as student teachers, should be offered orientation to their supervisorial and legal duties. They should also be familiarized with the policies and procedures established by the school and school district.

These considerations are important as schools strive to carry out their responsibility to protect the physical health and safety of their students. In recent years, however, educators have begun to realize that all aspects of the school environment affect the quality of education. Less tangible factors such as emotional and social climates can support or undermine educational objectives. Schools are total experiences for students and staff alike—what occurs both in and out of the classroom forms a seamless background that affects the well-being of all.

School Environments at Risk

Commitment to improving the school environment in all its aspects requires allocating resources and creating proper conditions to provide a supportive and healthy environment for youth. It also requires recognizing the potential and actual physical and social hazards that exist in the school, its surrounding community and the students' families.

Many of our inner-city urban schools are experiencing an unrelenting deterioration of their capacity to deliver education. Inner-city problems include:

- poverty
- widespread alcohol and other drug use
- violence
- unemployment
- youth gangs
- deteriorating housing
- closed businesses
- low educational attainment by parents
- teen pregnancies
- inadequate tax support for education and social and health services

These and other social factors combine to create formidable barriers to meeting the educational needs of children and youth. Despite technological and instructional advances in education, adverse circumstances and changes in significant parts of our society have diminished the capacity of far too many schools to provide the basic necessities that make education possible.

Inner-city schools, like all others, are total environments. School services, instruction and environment and the surrounding community are interrelated and have a significant impact on each other. Substantial social problems in various communities are reflected in the schools in those communities.

As discussed earlier, the first responsibility of the school is to provide a safe and healthy physical environment and protect students on their way from school and during the school day. Conditions in the inner-city environment make it increasingly difficult to meet this basic ethical and legal requirement. Schools have taken extraordinary steps to try to assure that this priority is achieved. However, because many inner-city communities lack basic safety for their citizens, these efforts have had only a limited success. Without this foundation, schools are inhibited from developing an atmosphere supportive of learning. Therefore, schools must establish basic levels of safety so students' attention can be devoted to the teaching/learning process.

School leaders can begin by making sure that unwanted outside influences are kept off of or removed from the school. The disruptive effects of outside influences such as drug dealing or gangs, can undermine campus authority. School authorities have the legal responsibility and the right to make sure that these unwanted groups are kept from school grounds. In some instances, these provisions extend to areas near the campus.

Disruptions at school, both in and out of the classroom, wreak havoc with education. Such disruptions must be dealt with in a swift and effective manner to remove the individual or individuals precipitating these disturbances. School officials must also take steps to establish an environment that respects education and the rights of youth to participate in the process without distraction. The campus should be free of drugs and weapons. Where drugs or weapons or other contraband are found, school officials must see that they are removed, along with those persons responsible for their presence.

To reinforce these measures, school officials should develop contacts with community agencies interested in and responsible for

The Importance of Healthy School Environments

services that will support a safe atmosphere for the school. They must also involve parent groups to gain feedback from and give information to parents about progress being made at school. Parents can help reinforce the policies and procedures developed to create a safe haven at school.

Once the basic provisions for safety have been established and a stable environment has been created, school leaders can attempt to expand health-promoting activities. For these efforts to work, all affected parties must be involved in the process under the solid, lasting leadership of school administrators. Consistency and commitment must be translated into the daily schedules and activities of the school and into the attitudes and behavior of teachers, staff and students.

These are time-consuming tasks. Because the social environment is constantly changing, there will be periods of progress and setbacks. Yet, without these procedures, the benefits of education will be lost to our youth in these schools.

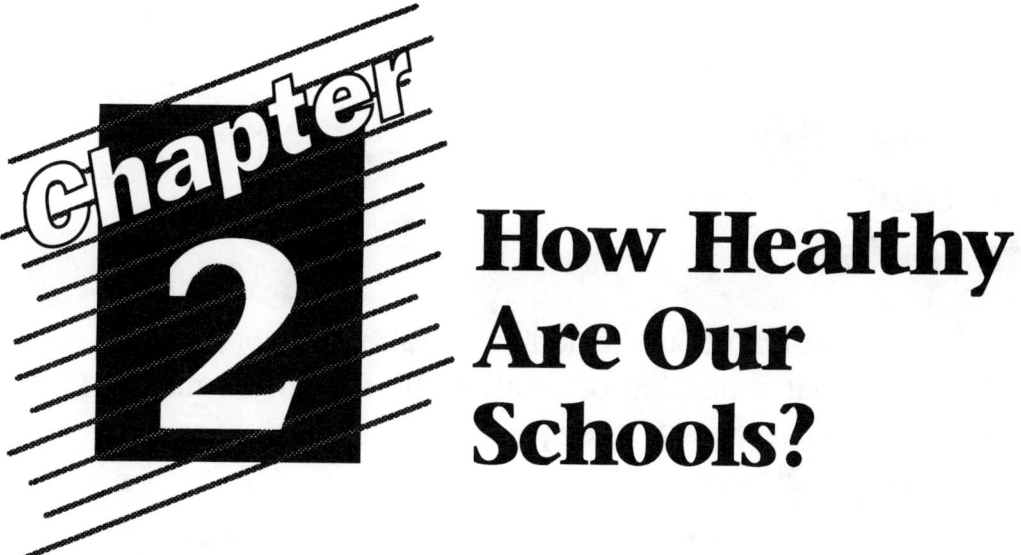

Chapter 2: How Healthy Are Our Schools?

THE HEALTH STATUS OF children and youth directly affects their ability to participate in school and to learn; educational achievement is related to health status. Health factors, including vision, hearing and behavioral dysfunctions, can affect the ability and willingness of children and youth to learn. In turn, health status is directly linked to educational status. National health statistics indicate that health status improves as the number of years of school completed rises. Lower education levels may lead to more health risks and poorer health status.

Schools have at least a two-fold role to play in promoting the health of students. First, schools have an obligation to be sure that their students have the basic health status that will enable them to learn. Second, schools can help to improve health status by reducing dropout rates and providing the skills and knowledge students need to participate fully in society.

How Healthy Are Our Students?

Much has been written about the declining health status of America's youth. The current generation of youth is the first in the nation's history to be less healthy than their parents, even though life expectancy continues to increase.

Children in our society appear to be moving in two different directions. One group is moving toward a healthier, better educated and higher socioeconomic status. For this group, data indicate a decline in death rates among children and youth and an improvement in overall indexes of health status and longevity.

These young people are in position to excel in society. They have high achievement test scores, suffer from less disease and fewer disabling conditions, are more physically fit and will have the opportunity to maintain or improve their socioeconomic status as they assume adult roles. The improvement of status for this group of youth has contributed to improved health statistics for the nation's children and youth as a whole.

However, a second group of children and youth presents a disturbing picture of an alarming decline in health status. The young people in this group are suffering from ever-growing risks to their well-being. Many of these risks stem from the circumstances of their births and their lives. Some of the most significant risks include:

- poverty
- inadequate health care coverage (related to poverty)
- inadequate diets
- sedentary lifestyles
- intended and unintended injury
- premature pregnancies
- school dropout rate

Deaths and Illness

According to the federal publication *Healthy People 2000* (U.S. Department of Health and Human Services, 1990) death rates for children decreased by 21 percent from 1977 to 1987. Death rates also declined for adolescents and young adults during this same period.

For children and adolescents, unintentional injuries are now the major cause of death. Most of these deaths are due to motor vehicle crashes. Although even these rates have been declining overall, largely due to mandatory safety seats for children and use of automobile safety belts, a disturbing upward trend has occurred for adolescents and young adults in recent years. Another fact of particular concern is the increase in the rates of child and youth homicide. Death by homicide has become the leading cause of death among Black males ages fifteen to nineteen.

Infectious and respiratory illnesses, although no longer the leading cause of death, remain problems for children and youth. Influenza and other respiratory diseases account for most of students' missed school days.

Chronic Conditions

Recent estimates of the prevalence of chronic health conditions for those under 18 years of age indicate that 31 percent, or almost 20 million children nationwide, have one or more chronic conditions. Of those with such conditions, 70 percent have one, 21 percent have two and 9 percent have three or more (Newacheck and Taylor, 1992).

Most children affected by these conditions report that their activities are not limited by the presence of the conditions most of the time. Respiratory allergies and repeated ear infections are the most commonly reported conditions. Other common chronic conditions include asthma, eczema and skin allergies, frequent or severe headaches, and speech defects.

Less common conditions include diabetes, sickle cell disease and cerebral palsy. Chronic conditions are more prevalent among boys than girls and among White children than Black children. The cumulative impact of these conditions on school attendance in 1988 resulted in 41 million absences.

Diet and Exercise Patterns

Diet and exercise patterns for our children and youth are changing. Youth are a less physically fit and fatter group. Between 1965 and 1985, skinfold thicknesses (a measure of body fat) of children increased. As measured by the U.S. Public Health Service, 15 percent of youth ages 12 to 19 were overweight in the 1976 to 1980 period.

Levels of fitness among youth in recent years have decreased, and the proportion of those leading sedentary lives has increased. Exercise is one of the most difficult health habits to influence. As overweight, unfit children grow into adulthood, they face increased risk of heart disease, cancer and stroke, the current leading causes of death among adults.

Poverty

According to the Maternal and Child Health Bureau of the U.S. Public Health Service, 12.6 million children under 18 years of age were living in poverty in 1989; this is almost 40 percent of the nation's poor. This represents an increase of 1 million since 1980. Slightly more than 20 percent of all children have no form of insurance coverage for health and medical services.

Black or Hispanic children are three times more likely to live in poverty than White children. Poverty contributes to many difficulties, including:

- learning disorders
- poor educational attainment

- higher drop-out rates
- inadequate nutrition
- more involvement with the criminal justice system
- psychological and emotional difficulties
- chronic physical conditions

Many children living in poverty live in two-parent families where both parents work. However, these parents cannot earn sufficient wages to keep their families out of poverty. The situation is complicated by parents' growing incapacity to achieve better jobs. In California, for example, the educational attainment of parents living in poverty has dropped over the past twenty years.

Two results follow. First, parents are limited in finding better-paying jobs. Second, parents' level of education often affects the level of education their children will achieve. Children living in poverty may remain there as they become adults with low education levels.

Poverty also puts children's health at risk. Children in poverty are less likely to see a physician. When they do see a doctor, it is more likely to be in a hospital than any other place. Children living in poverty spend nearly 60 percent more days in the hospital than those whose family income is above the poverty line. A similar pattern prevails for dental services.

Children without health insurance receive about half the care of those with health insurance. And this lack of care occurs when children are most vulnerable. It affects their schooling as well as their development. If the nation is to see substantial improvement in the health status of its children and youth, serious attention must be paid to the circumstances of daily living for disadvantaged children living in poverty.

Changes in Family Structure

Other changes in society have affected and will continue to affect school-age populations well into the next century. Working patterns for parents have changed. Fifty-four percent of mothers of children six to fourteen years of age are working outside the home either full- or part-time. Thirty-seven percent of mothers of children under the age of six are working outside the home. Teenagers are working as well: 45 percent work sixteen hours or more per week.

Family structure has also changed. In 1990, 15.9 million children, almost 25 percent of those under age 18, lived in families with only one parent. This percentage had more than doubled since 1970. Experts estimate that approximately 60 percent of all children will live with a single parent at some time prior to age 18. However, when remarriages are considered, 75 percent of children do live in two-parent households for at least some part of their youth.

A recent study indicates that children living with only one parent are less likely to finish school, particularly boys who live with their mothers. Nearly 40 percent of children live in single-parent households with less than $10,000 annual income. Black children are nearly three times as likely as White children to live with a single parent.

Other Changes

Other changes in society that have had and will continue to have an impact on education include the increased presence of other cultures, languages and ethnicities. In California schools, for example, by the year 2000, 42 percent of California children will be White, 36 percent Hispanic, 13 percent Asian, and 9 percent Black. Currently, one out of four California schoolchildren speaks a language other than English at home.

Other major metropolitan areas in the country are also experiencing this demographic shift. These changes have required schools to adapt their school schedules, curricula and relationships with parents and other family members.

How Healthy Are School Personnel?

Changes in the school-age population provoke much discussion and planning by state and local education agencies. However, looking only at students and their needs misses a substantial component of schools—administrators, teachers and other staff. Millions of teachers, administrators and other staff spend their working careers in American schools. As a group, school personnel are subject to the same rigors of life and challenges to health as other members of the workforce.

Schools are among the largest employers in the nation. According to 1988 statistics, more than 4.3 million people work in public school districts and schools in the nation. Add the slightly more than 539,000 employees in private elementary and secondary schools, and the total is almost five million school employees overall.

The qualifications and performance of school personnel are fundamental to education. Motivation and enthusiasm are important ingredients for student success. School personnel with high levels of absenteeism, poor morale, low expectations of themselves and students, and rapid rates of turnover help to create an environment detrimental to learning.

How Healthy Are Our Schools?

> ## Elementary and Secondary School Personnel
>
> **Public Schools:**
> - School district administrators and other employees: 69,000
> - Principals and assistant principals: 127,000
> - Teachers: 2,316,000
> - Teachers' aides: 356,000
> - Librarians: 49,000
> - Guidance counselors: 73,000
> - Support staff: 1,378,000
>
> **Private Schools:**
> - Principals and assistant principals: 37,000
> - Teachers: 353,000
> - Teachers' aides: 40,000
> - Librarians: 12,000
> - Guidance counselors: 9,000
> - Other professionals: 26,000
> - Other noninstructional staff: 54,000
>
> Source: Center for Education Statistics, U.S. Department of Education, 1990.

School personnel are subject to the same kinds of health experiences as other segments of the population, including cancer, heart disease and stroke, as well as dependence on alcohol or other drugs, obesity, adverse consequences of distress, and infectious diseases. Many of these diseases and conditions are related to behaviors that can be modified.

The following table summarizes some of the conditions that affect school employees. These statistics indicate that there is a significant amount of avoidable disease, disability and death among school personnel. The behaviors contributing to these statistics are acquired over time as part of lifestyle. The personal, family and social aspects of these conditions affect any intervention efforts.

Health Status of School Personnel

Exercise

- Only one in five exercises lightly to moderately (e.g., walking thirty minutes a day) five or more times in a given week. One in ten exercises seven or more times weekly.
- Fewer than one in ten exercises vigorously enough to produce cardiorespiratory fitness (i.e., twenty minutes of sustained activity three times per week).
- One in four does not participate in physical activity at all.

The benefits of light to moderate exercise include increased life expectancy; enhanced quality of life; prevention or management of high blood pressure, coronary heart disease, diabetes, osteoporosis and depression; and lower rates of colon cancer and stroke. Exercise may also be linked to reduced back injury, and many consider exercise essential to weight management and weight loss.

High Blood Pressure

- Almost one in three suffers from hypertension.

Overweight, lack of physical activity, and alcohol and sodium intake are linked to high blood pressure. High blood pressure is associated with half of the more than 1.2 million heart attacks and two-thirds of the strokes that occur annually.

(continued on next page)

How Healthy Are Our Schools?

Health Status of School Personnel
(continued)

Nutrition
- One in four is overweight.

Nutrition is associated with five leading causes of death: coronary heart disease, cancer, stroke, noninsulin dependent diabetes mellitus and atherosclerosis. Overweight may be a risk factor for high blood pressure, coronary heart disease, certain types of cancer, lack of physical fitness and diabetes.

Tobacco
- Twenty-nine percent smoke.

Smoking is associated with 40 percent of coronary heart disease deaths for those under age 65, 30 percent of all cancer deaths, and 87 percent of lung cancer deaths. Each employee who smokes costs an employer more than $4,600 annually in health care costs, absenteeism and lost productivity.

Alcohol
- One in ten is addicted to alcohol and nearly one in twelve has difficulty with alcohol.

Alcohol is associated with half of all homicides, suicides and motor vehicle crash fatalities. The annual economic cost of alcohol problems was estimated to be $70 billion in 1990.

Source: *Healthy People 2000*, U.S. Department of Health and Human Services, 1990.

Rising Health Care Costs

Schools face some difficult challenges as economic cycles affect their ability to meet educational needs. The health status of their personnel is one such challenge. Many schools and districts are discovering that the cost of recruiting and retaining teachers is becoming prohibitive.

The health of school personnel affects total compensation for teachers, administrators and staff. Health care costs for school personnel have become significant factors in school finance, just as these same expenditures have affected government, business and industry. Accordingly, conservation of human resources has become an important consideration for the well-being of education.

This need is due in part to the continuing societal phenomenon of rising health care costs. The United States spends approximately 12 percent of its gross national product on health care services. This percentage translates into more than $800 billion spent on health care services in 1991, and this upward trend is expected to continue.

Organizations faced with accelerating health care costs have changed their social contracts with employees. In the past, health insurance was one benefit provided by most large employers to their employees. Increasingly, this is no longer the case. Because of the cost factor, business and industry have begun to limit benefits by providing employees with choices. Employees can choose from among several benefit packages that cover some costs, but not all.

Schools are faced with the same concerns that businesses and industries have for providing a comprehensive package of benefits. School districts and schools have responded to rising health care costs by reviewing their capability to provide comprehensive health insurance benefits. Many districts have increased the number of part-time employees to save benefit costs. Other districts have passed along increased health care coverage costs to employees.

Altering employee benefits is one response to the unabated rise in health care costs. Another response is to look at the condition of employees and to determine if any improvement can be achieved. Many businesses and industries have adopted policies that are known to promote health, such as a smoke-free workplace. Cigarette smoking contributes significantly to sick-care costs and lower productivity, due to illnesses from smoking itself and illnesses such as colds or flu that are exacerbated by smoking.

The costs of recruiting new employees, voluntary employee turnover rates, costs for substitute employees and productivity measures are related to health matters. If surveys of employee attitudes toward the working environment are added to this information, a comprehensive profile of the health of the work environment should emerge. Studies have shown that as these indicators of health status are improved, health care costs can be stabilized or reduced while employee satisfaction and productivity rise.

Health Promotion for Staff— A Key to a Healthy Environment

Because qualified and dedicated personnel are key to education, preservation of their capabilities is paramount. Many schools use staff or professional development days to help staff upgrade their knowledge and instruction skills or to review the functioning of the facility. Similar attention should be given to the health of all school employees on a regular basis.

Programs directed toward improving employee health status accomplish two important aims. First, health care costs for schools stabilize, as do absenteeism and turn-over rates, and employee satisfaction and productivity increase. Second, because of the nature of educational interactions in and out of the classroom, healthy instructional messages are reinforced in the school environment for the benefit of students.

Health promotion for staff also contributes to an integrated approach to health promotion at the school. Health comes to be seen as an important aspect of creating a healthy, supportive climate for learning. Such integration promotes the value of individual worth and underscores the importance of a collective approach to improving the school environment.

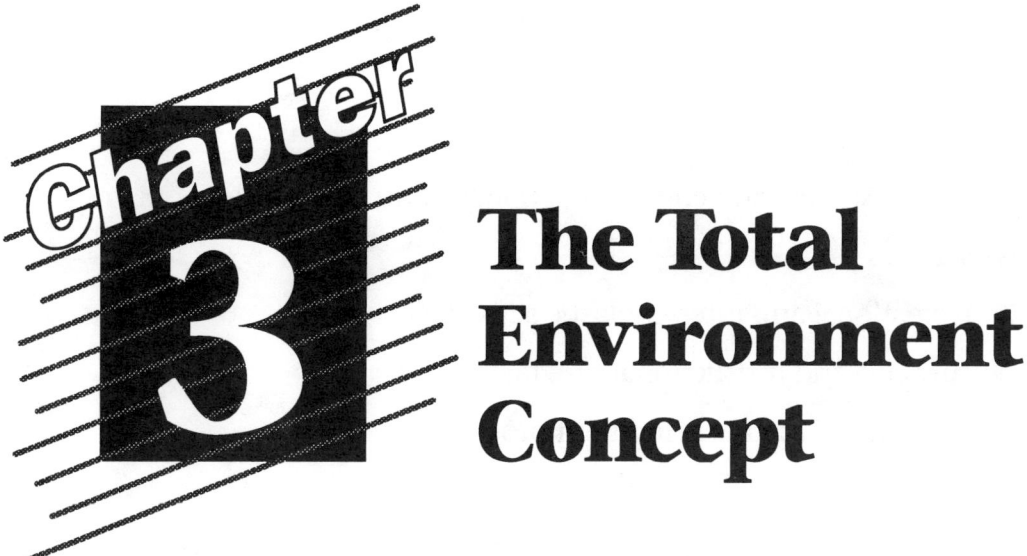

Chapter 3: The Total Environment Concept

SCHOOLS OCCUPY A PROMINENT place among American social institutions, and they have many opportunities to have a significant impact on the nation's quality of life. One such opportunity is to promote the health of everyone who goes to school daily. To do this, our view of the social and educational role of schools should be revised to incorporate a "total environment" perspective.

A total environment perspective takes the view that the physical, psychological and social dimensions of an organization are interdependent and interactive. As a school evolves, its work is changed by the accumulated experiences of those within it and the qualities of new students and personnel. Thus, the environment of an organization such as a school is influenced by the social context of which it is a part. In other words, schools are "open" systems, subject to many outside influences.

The total environment of the school includes:

- the school site and facilities, equipment and supplies
- student, teacher and staff interactions

The Total Environment Concept

- daily schedules
- administrative and educational policies and procedures
- services
- recreational and interscholastic activities
- curricula and instructional programs
- student and staff development programs

The environmental qualities of schools can be altered through a deliberate, planned process. Changes may be as simple as repainting classrooms, offices and hallways. They may involve designing staff development programs or organizing committees to identify and work on problems in the way the school functions on a daily basis. Or they may include substantive redesign and reequipment of the physical plant and grounds.

The school's physical environment and daily schedule may need to be adapted or modified to meet the needs of those who attend the school each day. As the school's physical plant and equipment ages and as characteristics of the surrounding community and students change, the need for altering the school environment in all its aspects becomes apparent.

The Culture of the School

All school experiences contribute to education. Schools help shape students' fundamental knowledge and skills and prepare them for adult roles. Most of the nation's attention has been focused on the curricular aspects of schools, i.e., reading, writing and arithmetic. Indeed, the largest proportion of school personnel are hired to teach. Yet schools exert many other complex and important influences.

School policies and procedures—the rules—and the way they are carried out play an important role in students learning how to get along in society. School rules may be very different from rules at home. Students are required to adapt to the school's environment. They quickly learn to pay attention to the rules, stated or unstated, that have priority, and to ignore the rules they understand to be irrelevant or unenforceable.

Students' contributions to the atmosphere of the school are influenced by their family, ethnic, linguistic and cultural backgrounds and their prior experiences in society and other schools. The backgrounds of school personnel also contribute significantly to the school's social environment. Teachers and other professional staff, particularly at the secondary level, have different disciplinary academic backgrounds and teaching responsibilities. This diversity influences the flow of the school day and the expectations, values and behavior of those who attend the school.

The interpersonal transactions that are part of the school day greatly affect the education of students and the careers of personnel. Students and school personnel create their own distinctive set of shared assumptions, beliefs, values and definitions of what the school is like and what roles and value they have in the school. These attributes are palpable but intangible products of the larger social environment and the interpersonal interactions within the school.

As students interact with each other and school personnel, the culture of the school is formed. This culture can be perceived as one participates in the daily life of the school. As participants, students and staff quickly learn their places in the school's environment and the value placed on their presence there. This kind of cultural learning can be positive or negative. It is affected by expectations created by prior experiences and also by the assumptions, beliefs and values that are reflected in the surroundings.

For example, what happens when students and school officials disagree on dress codes as a means of eliminating or minimizing the aura of gang presence on campus? Do school officials consult with

The Total Environment Concept

students and encourage their participation in the discussion? Or do school officials confer only among themselves and make their own decisions without consideration of students' opinions? How school administrators interact with others in the school gives a strong indication of the relative value and status of each group within the school.

What Does the Environment Communicate?

Large, impersonal physical plants can produce a sense of physical if not social isolation for young people. A similar observation may be made about the size of the school population. As school size increases, there is a greater chance that the individual student will become less important to the school.

The condition of the school's physical plant also transmits messages about the importance of students and staff members. Inner-city schools with high security fences, barred entrances and scarred buildings create a prison-like environment, where students merely exist for a period of time before they leave so that another group may enter. Staff in these institutions may be regarded, and may even regard themselves, as people who police and warehouse youth, rather than educators who are helping youth to acquire important knowledge and skills.

Policies and procedures greatly affect the social environment of the school and communicate a great deal about the way students and staff are valued. Students often have an "us-versus-them" mindset with regard to teachers and administrators. Disciplinary policies and other procedures may give credence to their feelings. If a school fails to address problems such as physical threats or alcohol and other drug use on campus, it reinforces students' alienation. Chronic teacher turnover, lack of enthusiasm in the classroom, excessive absenteeism, and lowered expectations for students all contribute to a poor social environment for learning. These conditions establish and reinforce the message to students that school is a difficult and unrewarding place.

We know that motivated students can and do learn despite adverse conditions, but a negative school environment is antithetical to student achievement. It delivers strong, negative messages about the value of schooling. Lower achievement and higher drop-out rates reflect poor conditions for learning in the classroom and school.

Evidence from schools and districts with high drop-out rates and low standardized test scores indicates that adverse school environment contributes to this lack of progress. Conversely, the success of some inner-city schools in promoting school achievement through policies and procedures, teacher/student interactions, and the improvement of the physical plant indicate that the school environment *can* be adapted to encourage learning, despite students' home and community conditions.

The Social Environment— A Crucial Component

Typical recommendations for improving school environment have encompassed the physical aspects of schools—the design and materials used for the school plant and the physical site for the buildings. But there is a second, equally important aspect of the school environment that must be considered. An understanding of the school's social climate—its source and the influences at work within it—is critical to any plan to improve the total environment.

The Total Environment Concept

> ### How Is Your School's Social Climate?
>
> - How much time and attention do teachers give students?
> - How enthusiastic are teachers in presenting their lessons?
> - What level of performance do teachers expect from students?
> - How are students treated individually and as a group?
> - Do teachers and administrators model the behaviors of responsible adults?
> - Do teachers and administrators follow through on their duties in the school outside the classroom?
> - Are student problems recognized and promptly handled, either directly or through referral?
> - Do teachers and administrators interact with students at school outside of their required duties?

Social Learning

Social experiences in the school setting help to shape students' attitudes, values and practices as they mature into adults. Children learn to adapt to the demands of varied social environments. An ability to adapt is increasingly necessary as children get older.

Social experiences contribute to the development of cognitive and behavioral skills important to success, as well as the social skills essential for coping with the social environment. These skills are learned in and out of the classroom, in school, at home and in the community. To cope with the many conflicting messages they receive, children must learn how to analyze situations, solve problems and make decisions. Our contemporary environment provides us with more information and social experiences than we can assimilate. Given this massive amount of information and experience, we develop systems for acquiring, sorting, evaluating and incorporating useful intelligence to manage our daily lives. Beliefs, internal standards, perceptions of the environment, prior experiences, rewards and punishments help us create these systems.

The ability to make decisions to ignore, keep or discard various input begins with early socialization experiences at home. It is augmented, refined and extended through experiences in the community and at school. The family instills values, beliefs and standards of permissible and impermissible behaviors. The family also imparts important attitudes and practices about health—nutrition, personal hygiene, coping with illnesses, and protective behaviors (e.g., wearing safety belts and immunization against diseases).

These messages are either reinforced or refuted by the school and community. School supplies technical knowledge and skills that elaborate on or refine earlier messages and help students develop behaviors important to full participation in society. Yet, as individuals, we quickly learn to discern the degree of consistency between messages and the way they are conveyed. Youth expect and have a great need for consistency between message and messenger.

Conflicts and Consistency

Conflicting demands and expectations of home and school often produce stressful situations for students. Health issues are particularly sensitive. There are many areas of potential conflict among home, school and community regarding health behaviors, including the following:

- personal hygiene
- nutrition
- tobacco, alcohol and other drug use
- family life and human sexuality
- use of health products, services and information

Conflict between the school's social environment and the messages taught in the classroom is of particular concern—for example, when the food available at school does not match the principles of healthy nutrition taught in class. School learning experiences designed to improve nutritional habits are unlikely to be incorporated as a value or as a behavior when school meals and snacks negate the educational message. Likewise, attempts to promote vigorous physical activity have little effect when there is little support by the school for regular physical exercise.

A less obvious but equally important conflict has to do with teachers' behavior and how their behavior is perceived by students. Surveys of student opinions of the health habits of teachers reveal that young people overestimate the prevalence of teachers who smoke, for example. Does the social environment of most schools make it appear that more adults smoke than is actually the case?

Because schools have areas in which staff smoke and because films and television often portray cigarette smoking as pervasive, young people consistently and substantially overestimate the prevalence of smoking among adults. This perception reinforces student impressions that smoking is a low-risk activity and a symbol of adult behavior. Youth are thus more likely to experiment with and become dependent upon tobacco. Over 90 percent of those who smoke began before age 18.

Other health habits exhibited by teachers, such as level of fitness, quality of diet and degree of overweight, may not differ much from students' perceptions. Students also observe other things about their teachers that may or may not be attributed to health factors. These include the number of teacher absences, enthusiasm for teaching, respect for students and others at school, and concern about the work environment.

Students have more difficulty observing the behavior and attitudes of school personnel other than teachers because they have little contact with them. However, the influence of these personnel may be transmitted to students through teachers and through out of classroom and extracurricular activities. Does this mean that those who come into contact with students each day—teachers, administrators and staff (to say nothing of parents and peers)—must be exemplary in their health behavior? Perhaps.

The Importance of Models

Much learning is done indirectly, through observation. We acquire needed knowledge, attitudes, values and skills as we witness the activities of others and the consequences of their actions. Youth who are able to see behaviors and their rewarded consequences learn valuable lessons without having to use time-consuming and costly trial-and-error methods to arrive at the same end.

Observation enables us to model behaviors perceived to be useful. Observed behavior is internalized and may eventually be expressed by the observer. This process is quite complex and not fully understood. However, we do know that the amount of attention paid to a behavior varies according to the attention commanded by or the perceived importance of the individual who models the behavior.

Teachers and other school officials have a great deal of potential influence, because they occupy positions of power and importance in the school. Students extend this recognition beyond official school duties to other aspects of life, as their frequent requests to teachers for advice attest. Teachers' influence extends to appearances (both physical and social), attitudes and health behaviors that students observe.

School officials and teachers can be important role models. Their stature helps lend them credibility in the eyes of young people when social environments may be conflicting and ambiguous. In these situations, the more overt and generalized aspects of adult authority figures are what are noticed and judged—their general appearance, speech, style, age, symbols of success or status, and established or apparent expertise.

Young people are very vulnerable to influences that they would imitate. As children, youth take their cues from older and authoritative adults at home and in school. These figures are perceived as reliable guides to proper behavior. However, as youth move into adolescence and begin to shed childish identities and acquire adult roles, they look at adult authority figures differently. This process may be accelerated through media influences and the feedback youth experience when they try to mimic adult behaviors.

Adolescence stimulates youth to develop their own identities and modes of functioning without the assistance of traditional authority figures. They often turn to their own or somewhat older peers as guides to this process. Peers are important role models in adolescence, as well as in other periods of development. Unfortunately, peers are often in the same situation as their observers. They, too, are trying to sort out how to think, feel and perform—a process filled with trial and error for all involved.

Young people, as well as adults, are attracted to individuals who have an aura of confidence and authority. They are also attracted to those who have apparent success in appealing to youth. Teachers and other school officials may be able to influence youth if they have good interactions with young people in and out of the classroom or if they possess qualities with which young people identify. These qualities may relate to the relative youth or youthful appearance of a teacher; a teacher's gender or ethnicity; or his or her involvement with extracurricular activities in or out of school.

People come from different backgrounds with different experiences and expectations, and behaviors and their consequences are not always seen. Adults at the school are more likely to be influential role models if they share the background and characteristics of the student body of the school. Interest and concern about young people will also make them more attractive to youth, as will conducting themselves in ways that indicate they are fair-minded and reliable.

None of these qualities necessarily affect what teachers teach, but they do affect the way adults at the school conduct themselves in and out of the classroom and how they handle their interactions with students and others in the school. Adults who serve as role models can give reassurance to adolescents during a turbulent time of life as well as to young children during formative years.

Messages That Support Health

Students recognize the similarities and differences between what adult authority figures present in and out of the classroom and the way they conduct themselves in the social environment of the school. Those in a position to teach about health topics are most vulnerable to students' comparisons between what is said and what is practiced. But role-modeling messages must also be supported by others in the school environment to be effective. To focus on a single individual—teacher, administrator or student—puts an unfair and unreasonable emphasis on one individual's responsibility for others' health choices.

Naturally, part of our message in supporting health is to encourage individuals to take control over areas where they can act in healthful ways. But it is often difficult for children and youth as well as adults to see how the social environment matches up with messages given in the classroom. For example, students have every right to question health messages about smoking when they see that cigarettes are widely and legally available. In addition, cigarette makers sponsor any number of athletic and cultural events; the federal government supports tobacco farming; and smoking is allowed almost everywhere, including homes and schools (although this is changing).

The fact that the teacher with the antismoking message does not smoke plays only a small role in youths' understanding of the use of tobacco in society. When wider societal actions match antitobacco messages, the modeled behavior and message are more strongly substantiated. As more social environments become smoke free, including the school, students will come to see that health messages against the use of tobacco are to be taken seriously.

Health messages are up close and personal. Such messages are evaluated by students as they examine their own current behaviors and observe the behaviors of others. When disparities are found, students may question the credibility of health advocates. Youth may not be ready to make a thoughtful evaluation of the social environment and other factors that contribute to or compromise health. This tendency is natural in a society that extols the importance of individual choice and the right to self-determination. However, we must also consider how the physical and social environments shape one's opportunities for self-determination.

Tales of personal successes against obstacles found in society, whether economic, social or educational, are often used to illustrate the idea that the grit and determination of the individual will overcome all barriers. As educators, we know that these stories help to stimulate and motivate individuals to achieve. At the same time, we also know that there are key ingredients for successful adult lives.

Among these key ingredients is success in school, which translates into opportunities for success in life. There is a continuity between supportive home environments, school successes and successful adult roles. Conflicts between home, school and community lead to decreased opportunities. The capacity of individuals for growth and development can be heavily influenced by social circumstances.

Commitment— A Key Ingredient

The school environment will reflect society's many inconsistencies and contradictions about health practices. But we can help students avoid the unnecessary and tragic consequences of poor health habits by making the social environment match up with health messages as much as possible. This does not mean that everyone in school must mindlessly follow a prescribed regimen of behavior, nor does it mean that there will be only one correct way for staff to behave. It does, however, require a commitment by school leaders to provide a supportive environment to protect and promote the health of students and staff.

Our society is as healthy as it wants to be, according to the noted economist Victor Fuchs. We determine how healthy we are by our collective and individual actions. To improve health status, we must reallocate scarce resources and apply them to health.

The school is a micro-economy of resources. Fiscal, physical, personnel and time resources can be used for many things, among them improving the health of students and staff. When we reshuffle existing resources by redefining and redesigning the social environment of the school and make its physical environment match and reflect its improved social environment, the odds for developing healthy graduates and a healthy staff are improved appreciably.

Chapter 4
Partnerships for Change

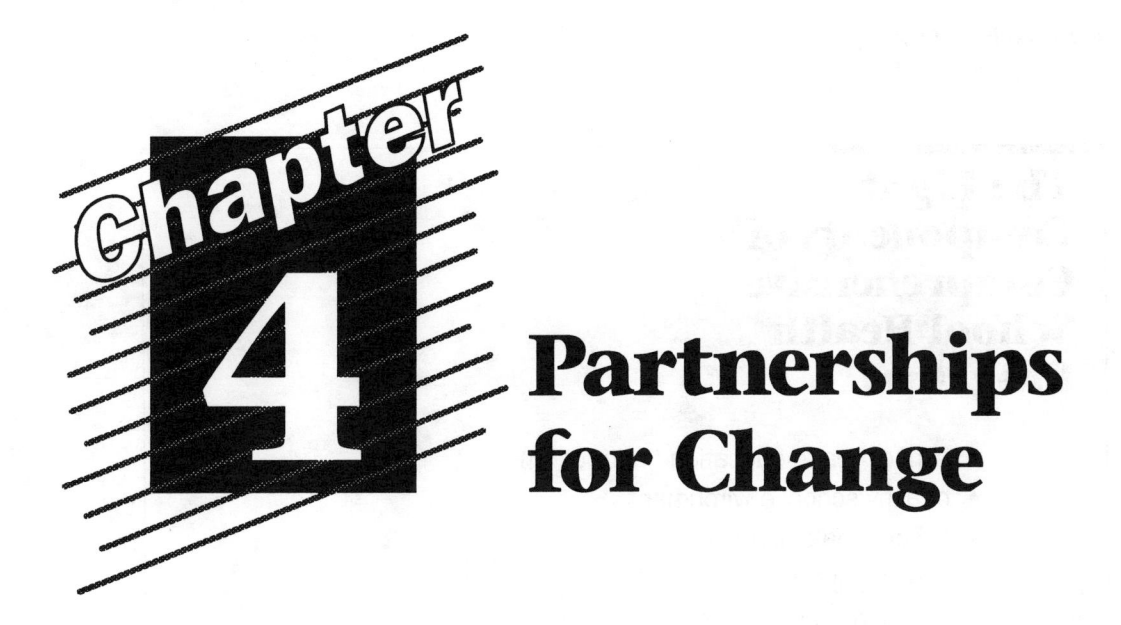

A COMPREHENSIVE SCHOOL HEALTH program provides a foundation for making schools healthy and successful. Schools have eight components that, when planned and implemented on an integrated basis, can support and promote the health of students and staff alike. These include school health services, health instruction and healthy school environment.

Development of these components into a comprehensive school health program requires leadership from within the school as well as from the community. Administrative leadership can provide direction for the program and emphasize the importance of health. School leaders can tap the personnel and physical resources of the school to develop the program.

The Eight Components of Comprehensive School Health Programs

- school health education (instruction)
- healthy school environment
- school health services
- school physical education
- school nutrition and food services
- school-based counseling and personal support
- schoolsite health promotion
- school, family and community health promotion partnerships

Adapted from D. D. Allensworth and L. J. Kolbe. 1987. The Comprehensive School Health Program: Exploring an Expanded Concept. *Journal of School Health* 57 (10): 409–412.

Teachers, administrators, other staff and students should be involved in the planning, implementation and evaluation process to ensure that the program is relevant and timely. Community agencies can be tapped to provide important support, if not direct services. Official and voluntary health agencies, national, state and local health care providers organizations, local business and industry and service clubs can be counted upon to make contributions to the school. Partnerships for health are an excellent idea and quite feasible. The current environment for education encourages such partnerships, from special instructional programs to tutoring to acquiring teaching materials and equipment.

Content Areas for Comprehensive Health Education

Children and youth need to acquire basic knowledge and skills to protect their health and that of others. The following list indicates the typical content areas for instruction.

- family life
- nutrition
- mental/emotional health
- personal health
- substance use and abuse
- prevention and control of disease
- consumer health
- injury prevention and safety
- community health
- environmental health

A comprehensive school health program will be reflected in the physical, emotional and social aspects of the school. The "feel" of the school will change as strategies for making the school a healthier place to be become part of the rhythm and functions of the school day. As the planning and implementation activities for the instructional aspect of a school health program have their impact, school policies and procedures, daily schedules and expectations of students and staff will change. One of the beneficial effects of a comprehensive school health program is an altered view of the role of the school among those who study and work there. Such a program also enhances consideration of and respect for each individual.

Partnerships for Change

Because of the interactive nature of educational settings and their influence on social learning, all those involved in schools have a part in helping achieve better health for the institution. Administrators, teachers, other staff, students, parents and outside groups interested in the well-being of schools, and in health specifically, all have a role to play.

Key Roles at the School

Because of the interdependent nature of school environments, school personnel must be involved in or support required changes in physical and social conditions affecting the environment. Most particularly, those who have the greatest influence on their colleagues and on students must be involved in change. These key actors must be part of any endeavor to alter the culture and direction of the school toward health. Such efforts may be personally rewarding and have substantial measurable benefits in the future.

Administrators

Administrative leadership is an important ingredient in the effort to make schools healthy and productive. Such goals can be difficult to achieve in a societal atmosphere that continually demands more from schools. Schools have more competing demands for their resources than they can accommodate. If scarce human, physical and time resources are to be reallocated toward initiating a healthy school environment, school administrators must see health as a priority.

Schools do not have enough physical space, personnel and time to address all worthy ideas and suggestions. Administrators, from the district level to the individual schools, must make important decisions about the allocation of scarce educational resources. Although health is a foundation for school success, it is often considered the responsibility of the family, community and, ultimately, the individual. Administrators who adopt this view are unlikely to allocate resources to health education.

Some administrators may themselves be at high risk for health problems because of their lifestyles or health behaviors. They may be reluctant to get involved in health promotion programs. Of course, if these administrators become convinced of the personal health threat of their lifestyles, they may be willing to make personal changes that could be incorporated into the school schedule.

As leaders of the school, administrators play a crucial role in the assessment of the school climate and how the results of such assessment are interpreted to students, staff, parents and the community. Administrators must be able to articulate how any changes toward a healthier climate meet existing traditions and expectations. Leadership must provide direction and commitment for change and a process that will enable change to occur in a manner consistent with the characteristics of the school, its student body and its staff.

Administrators must pay attention both to the achievement of specific, measurable goals and objectives and to the interpersonal qualities of school life. Clearly specifying the expectations for students and staff and providing a supportive environment to help them meet these expectations combines humanistic and achievement orientations. Leadership includes implicitly and explicitly acknowledging and valuing the contributions of teachers, aides, counselors, support staff and students.

Administrators are key actors in conceiving a plan to create a healthier school environment and implementing the activities that result from the concept. Administrators stand to benefit personally from participating in health-promoting activities as well as to gain professionally through the improved performance of the school.

Teachers

Teachers are crucial to any health promotion plan at the school because they spend the most time with students. Students are learning not only from the curricula and the lessons designed by faculty to develop knowledge and skills, but also from the way teachers present themselves in both the classroom and the general environment of the school. School personnel, particularly teachers, have to accept and adopt health promotion programs and changes in the environment to a great extent before any benefits for youth can be seen.

Teacher attitudes and practices expressed in interactions with students have the potential to reinforce powerful health messages. Health promotion programs can improve teacher health status and morale, and this benefits both teachers and their students. Healthy teacher role models help reinforce to students that health is instrumental to leading a satisfying and productive life.

Obviously, teachers must be involved in every step of the change processes. Their interactions with students and their commitment to proposed changes are vital to making health promotion programs work. Teachers should participate from the beginning phases of program development to the implementation and evaluation. Teacher responses to improvements in the social climate have a critical effect on the diffusion of change throughout the school.

Teachers often think that they don't have much power, yet they have a group of growing and developing young people in front of them each day. Because of their positions and expertise, teachers have a great deal of authority, which transcends the classroom. Change must engage teachers in a serious, involved way to optimize the benefits gleaned from an improved school environment.

Other School Staff

Other school staff support the teaching/learning process by linking the various activities of the school. To a large extent, school staff are responsible for making sure that the school's physical environment and services, including instructional resources, are well maintained and function properly. Without services such as food services, environmental sanitation, safety provisions, communicable disease control, and vision and hearing screening, schools would not be able to act in the best interests of students, teachers and parents.

Therefore, support staff should be included in any planning process to promote health at the school. Support staff are important to the school's bottom line as well as its productive capability. Support staff can facilitate health promotion programs by helping to modify schedules so that facilities will be available or by making sure the environment reflects priorities for health. For example, support staff may be responsible for making sure that equipment used for fitness activities is maintained, that fire extinguishers and emergency systems are functioning, or that food service reflects health priorities and is tailored to the tastes of students and staff.

Students

To be effective, education needs students who are both willing and able to learn. When their basic health needs are not met, students will not be able to learn. Our society is increasingly unable to provide basic medical and health services for youth. An increasing number of young people are living in families below the poverty line. This situation raises great concerns that children and youth at school are less able to take advantage of educational programs.

Furthermore, students are sensitive to their environments and quick to observe discrepancies between what is taught in the classroom and what is practiced in school, home and community. Students come to school with important family and community beliefs, values and practices, all of which form a foundation of experiences that affect their response to educational transactions. Changes in the school environment to improve health have the potential to act as influential models for students' attitudes and behavior.

Changes in the way students are approached and how the school day is structured are significant occurrences. Students are likely to be the group most affected by such changes in the school environment. They will have to adapt as health promotion programs become a more prominent part of their school experiences. Students need to be able to make connections between these programs, health instruction messages, behavior of school personnel, and how health behavior is modeled at home.

Accordingly, students need to be involved with health promotion as part of their school day, including:

- health instruction in the classroom
- fitness activities
- health protection through health services
- supportive food services
- a physical environment
- a school atmosphere that promotes respect and dignity for all

Students need to participate in making sure that their school environments provide these health promotion services and reflect these qualities. They should also be given responsibility and authority for ensuring that their needs are being met. Students can be given the opportunity to participate through organized student government, which has a defined relationship with school administrators. Students should also be included in a school health council made up of teachers, health educators, nurses, administrators and other school personnel.

A drawback to including students in the process, however, is the frequent division between school personnel and students. Often students believe that they are in an "us-versus-them" situation. To the extent that this barrier exists, it substantially affects the role-model influence of teachers and other school staff. Thus, when changes in school personnel occur as a result of a health promotion program, students may not interpret the changes in the intended way.

However, when teaching/learning transactions, environmental changes, parental and community involvement and student involvement are combined, the inevitable effects of changes cannot be ignored. Misinterpreted, perhaps, but not ignored. Eventually, the weight of change and the greater consistency between the educational messages given and the reinforcement provided within the school environment will have a positive influence on students.

School Board Members

School board members have the legal responsibility for the school district. Board members come from the communities served by the school and typically have children in school. Board members come from all walks of life, with varying attitudes and experiences in education as well as health.

Because of their legal duties, board members have considerable influence over general and specific matters pertaining to schools. They make budgetary and programmatic decisions affecting the broad spectrum of schools in their communities. Environmental improvement and health promotion initiatives have the potential to involve many people, both in and out of the schools. They also have implications for medical care benefit savings and working conditions. Therefore, board members should be involved in developing such programs. Changes to one school's environment will probably be appropriate for other schools in the district.

Support from board members can be translated into superintendent and school administrator support. While this is no guarantee of success in and of itself, the imprimatur of the school board can serve as a catalyst for reallocating resources through systematic planning and for involving parents and community groups outside the school as part of the process.

Building Partnerships for Change

There are many ways individuals and groups outside of the school can contribute to improving the school environment. Building partnerships between the school and community is essential to the long-term success of any schoolsite health promotion program.

Parents

Parental support for any proposed changes in the school environment is very important. Parents play a fundamental role in helping their children learn how to function in society. Family health beliefs, knowledge, attitudes and practices are powerful models for children's behavior. When the messages from home and school are consistent, there will be fewer difficulties between parents and the school.

Parents are responsible, morally and legally, for ensuring that their children's health needs are met. Although parental participation in the school is desirable, it is not always available. Nevertheless, parents need to understand how their children adapt to the school environment and how their values and priorities for their children are similar to or different from what the young people experience in school. If they realize how their attitudes, values and behavior are used as models by their children, parents can work with the school to help their children adjust to differences between the messages and climate of the school and those of the home and community.

As schools see the need for change, school personnel must actively involve parents in the planning process. Many important health values and behaviors are developed at home, and any proposed school program is quite likely to affect them. Even when the school is not contradicting parents, it is important for parents to know of and support programs.

Parents are in a crucial position to reinforce learning acquired at school. In turn, parents would like to know that the school supports and reinforces their health beliefs, attitudes and practices. Parents may want to become part of programs to improve school environments at the schoolsite. Parents often volunteer in elementary classrooms to support teachers. Parents may also participate at school because they have particular expertise in a certain area of a school program. Parents may be involved in parent/teacher or home and school organizations. These organizations can be of great help in identifying and gathering resources to meet particular needs.

The active involvement of parents helps build bridges between home and school. Parental involvement can help make programs a success. Organized into groups, parents can provide advice, information and feedback to school personnel. Parents may also want to become program participants with their children or separately in one or more health promotion activities.

All of these types of involvement help to build solid support for environmental changes and health promotion at the school. After all, students learn most of their health habits and develop their view of the role of health in life through their home environments. Through cooperative interaction with the school, parents are in a pivotal position to reinforce the healthy behaviors and skills learned at school.

Community Organizations

In addition to parental involvement, schools are being encouraged to form partnerships with community organizations to support academic programs and extracurricular activities. Successful partnerships have worked to improve the quality of school life, from additions to the library and computer equipment to opportunities for students to refine and extend their education.

Community agency partnerships take advantage of the long tradition school health programs have of involving the community in protecting and promoting health at school. Outside groups have always had a role to play in helping the school to become a healthier environment. For example, as budget cuts lead to the loss of many school-based health services, official health agencies have been used to fill gaps for screening and other services. Many local and national health agencies enhance school health programs by offering age-appropriate classroom materials and guest speakers on a variety of topics. Professional health, medical and dental organizations are also interested in the health of children and youth. They can be called on to assist in tasks from forming public policy and conducting research to providing educational services in the classroom.

Private industry has been the most recently featured outside group to form partnerships with schools to improve educational programs. Many companies have participated in the schools by providing resources to meet specific health needs as well as equipment for education, including health promotion. Similarly, community service clubs have had a long tradition of supplying certain items, such as eyeglasses, which can facilitate learning and help children adapt to school.

Concerned individuals from the community can also make a difference. For example, the "I Have A Dream" Foundation was set up by a businessman in New York. He visited the elementary school from which he had graduated and promised the sixth graders there that if they would finish school he would guarantee their college expenses.

Other outside groups with an interest in promoting health include parent/teacher organizations and youth groups. Parent/teacher organizations have the opportunity to view the school from a close yet different perspective than that of those directly involved in the daily activities of the school. They are in an excellent position to identify needs and help reconcile differences between the environments of the school, home and community. Populations of youth groups are selected from the schools. These groups provide young people valuable experiences and offer them opportunities to apply health messages learned at school.

Schools are highly visible public entities. They attract a great deal of attention for what they do or don't do, or for what happens at school, good and bad. Even though schools are legally separate from the communities in which they are located, community people and agency representatives often express their interest in or concern about what is happening at the schools.

To promote health and protect the environment at school, school officials are well advised to include community members when changes are being considered. Involvement by the community in the process of planning change builds trust, openness and commitment to whatever change takes place.

Often such involvement is resisted because it adds an extra burden of organizing, communicating and processing. Community members may not readily understand the constraints and objectives of schools; they may require special training. Also, they may not participate in ways typical of school populations. Many reasons can be used to justify resisting the involvement of the community in planned school change processes. However, these reasons should not eliminate community participation. Ample evidence indicates that community members will participate in school affairs whether or not they are invited.

What happens at school is of interest to many in the community who do not have children in school. Those who do have children in school may be even more interested. Schools should take advantage of the interest and energy in the community to help facilitate school improvements. Commitment to the school and to change can more easily be achieved by involving community members; doubts, suspicions and demands for accountability can be allayed, if not eliminated, by including community members.

The time and effort needed are well worth the investment when costs of answering potentially hostile opponents are considered. Furthermore, involvement of community members presents opportunities for developing networks of resources that, in time, may yield bonuses for the school beyond anything imagined.

Partnership Resources

Local Resources

City or county health departments	Service clubs
Hospitals	County/district offices of education
Community coalitions	Parents and parent groups
School support groups	Students and student organizations
Voluntary health agencies	Health professionals
Business and industry	

State Resources

Educational agencies	Interest groups
Public health agencies	Trade associations
Health insurance companies and associations	Professional organizations

National Resources

Official education agencies	Medical and dental professional associations
Education professional associations	Interest groups
Public health agencies	Health insurance companies and associations
Public health professional associations	Trade associations

Chapter 5
Schoolsite Health Promotion

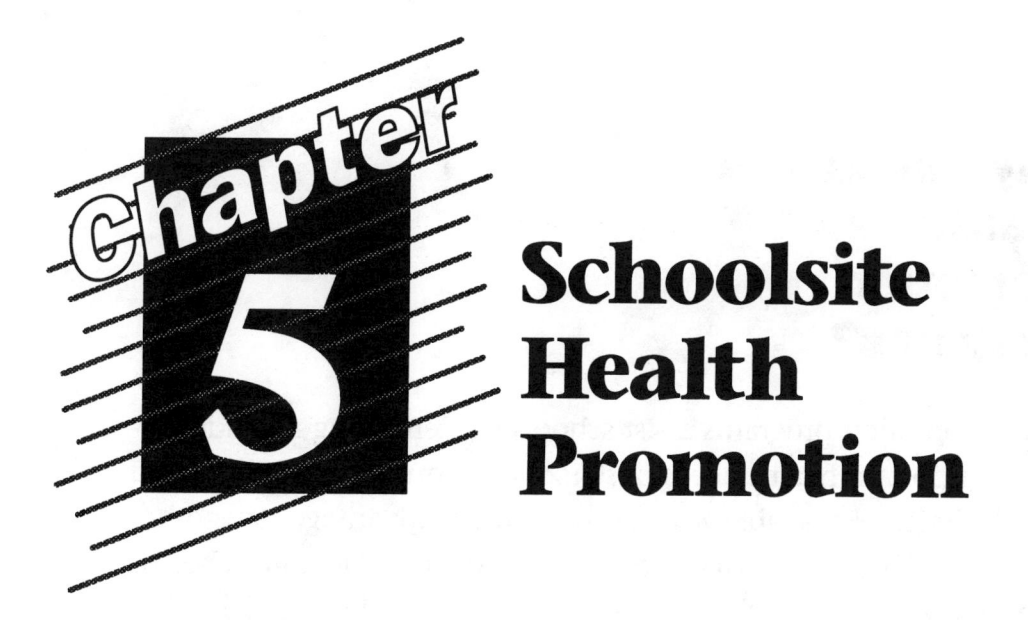

HEALTH PROMOTION HAS HAD numerous definitions. For our purposes, health promotion is comprised of planned learning opportunities that help school staff adopt healthy behaviors. There are many activities included within health promotion, such as smoking cessation, weight reduction and dietary changes, stress management and physical fitness. While many of these individual activities have been happening in schools for some time, the combination of these efforts within a planned context with specific goals and objectives is something new. Because schools are numerous, are found throughout our society and employ millions of people, they are logical and desirable sites for health promotion activities.

Why Schoolsite Health Promotion Programs?

Health promotion programs assist schools in identifying and addressing the important health needs of school personnel. The facilities and trained personnel available at schools give them advantages over other worksites in developing health promotion programs. Organized health promotion in the schools can achieve the same benefits found in other worksites, including improved productivity, decreased absenteeism, improved morale and lower health care costs. These beneficial changes for school personnel also affect the teaching/learning process. Motivated, healthy school personnel are better able to arouse and maintain the interest of students in any subject area.

Health promotion and disease prevention programs at the school worksite take positive and affirmative action to assist employees to take control over their health. Programs focus on reducing risks for disease and improving productivity and job satisfaction. Employers have increasingly recognized that organized programs of health enhancement—from stress management to weight reduction to smoking cessation—provide a return on investment for the costs of such programs, aside from savings on sick care costs.

Adults have the opportunity to protect and improve their health status by practicing behaviors that are consistent with good health. Lifestyle changes can help people avoid most of the leading causes of death and disability. Clear evidence demonstrates that health and lifestyle are linked. There has been a 40 percent reduction in coronary heart disease deaths and a 50 percent decline in stroke deaths since 1970. These reductions were achieved largely through reduced rates of cigarette smoking, lower average blood cholesterol levels, and increased control over high blood pressure. Deaths from motor vehicle crashes also declined almost 30 percent since 1970, primarily due to lower rates of alcohol use, increased safety belt use and lower speed limits.

Key Ingredients for Successful Programs

These developments are encouraging, but American patterns of living still produce results that may hinder further progress and escalate health care costs, loss of productivity, absenteeism and premature death. Changing lifestyle patterns is a complicated process, but several key ingredients can greatly aid health promotion efforts at the school.

Administrative Leadership

An essential requirement for successful schoolsite health promotion and environmental improvement is the enthusiastic and wholehearted support of the school's administrator. Time after time, attempts to improve health programs in schools have failed, primarily due to lack of commitment on the part of school administration.

In many schools, the top administrator wields a great deal of authority and influences the psychological and social climate of the school, as well as its physical aspects. Priorities of school administrators become priorities for all those at school. Each school has its distinctive character, which is a reflection, at least in part, of its leader.

Leadership is challenged to envision and articulate goals and objectives for the school as they relate to the district and state mandates and community standards. Articulation of goals and objectives occurs in the policies and procedures established for the conduct of the school day; the expectations held of students, faculty and staff; and the physical and social climate of the school. A school climate that provides support for useful communications and reflects commitment to education and to improving the conditions for learning will implicitly and explicitly express respect for and acknowledge the importance of staff and faculty, as well as students. These elements help establish an atmosphere for productive change.

Enthusiasm by school leadership is often missing in the equation for environmental improvement. When this occurs, change is possible, but is less likely to be significant. Programs will take much longer to develop and implement, and will be subject to elimination should any adverse conditions arise. Proposals to change physical and social climates and introduce health promotion programs may appear to be too involved and costly, in human and material terms. Leaders may be pressed to accomplish the goals and objectives of education in a climate of declining budgets and deteriorating morale of students, faculty and staff, and a community environment critical of schools because of the many problems in education. If administrative support is not present, those with a commitment to improving the environment must assess the probability of success. Efforts to educate and persuade leadership to make changes may be a lengthy process.

Support and Participation

If administrative support is present but the target audiences for environmental change are indifferent to any proposed program, a great deal of planning and implementation effort can be exerted without results. It may do more harm than good to insist that a program be adopted regardless of interest.

Unwarranted and unwanted intrusions into the daily lives of people at the school may alienate them. Further damage is done when the costs of developing unwanted programs are calculated. Subsequent proposals will be judged according to past experiences. In addition, without sufficient numbers enrolled in programs, any evaluation would reveal a paucity of participation, which would not support continuation.

Conversely, enthusiastic support by students, faculty, staff and administrators, as well as parents and community members, demonstrates a commitment to making changes, establishing both need and interest for programs. Such interest may represent pent-up demand. It may also represent careful and thorough assessment and planning that involves the target audiences for change.

Participation in new endeavors is often dependent upon the degree to which target audiences have had the opportunity to participate in identifying needs and interests, establishing priorities, and planning the program. Participation in program development builds commitment as people gain specific programmatic benefits from their involvement. Enthusiasm is reinforced when programs are offered in times, locations and formats that are compatible with people's responsibilities and daily activities. Making programs as widely available as possible also contributes to support for change.

Lastly, interest is often stimulated by programs that are relatively rapid responses to stated needs, regardless of their merit for health-related reasons. For example, simply changing paint or color schemes within the school can have a profound effect on mood and attitude.

Respect

Another essential ingredient of success is respect for the goals and objectives of the proposed program. Respect is derived from at least two sources. One is a generalized climate of respect for the dignity, value and worth of all in the school. This climate is developed by leadership, at least initially. Sustaining respect throughout the school then becomes the responsibility of all at the school. The personal influence and authority of school leaders in modeling appropriate behavior is as important as the implementation of policies and procedures in a respectful manner.

Respect is also derived from the care and consideration given to individual concerns and ideas as expressed through alteration and adaptation of the school environment. Serious attention given to the conditions that make the working and educational environment better are appreciated by all involved. Involvement is a key corollary to establishing and maintaining respect. Respect is facilitated by open, clear communication that allows information and needs to be passed freely through the organizational hierarchy.

Communication

Developing school health programs requires frequent and multilevel communications among students, staff and administrators. Because of the different responsibilities, roles and expectations and the involvement of outside influences in the school, communications are particularly important.

Inclusion in formal and informal information loops provides staff and students with the understanding that they are important parts of the organization. Communications must not only be from the top down but from the bottom up, as well as lateral. Communication is made easier when the important health reasons for changing the environment and providing health promotion programs are translated into terms that are meaningful and useful to all involved. Discussions should allow for presentation of both the current state of affairs in the school as well as opportunities to express what should be occurring in the school.

Formal communications, such as newsletters and bulletins, allow important information needed by everyone to be distributed. Informal communications allow people to address important concerns at the level and point where interaction, problem solving and decision making are timely.

All parties involved should offer feedback to the leadership of the school on ways to improve programmatic offerings and environmental conditions. Without systematic as well as random feedback, it is difficult to assess the acceptability, utility, value and relevance of any organizational changes, especially in health promotion. A feedback system allows for continual reassessment of important aspects of the school environment. It also allows for evolutionary changes as educational priorities, school staff, student and family characteristics, and community qualities shift.

Staff Development

Staff development opportunities must be considered a key ingredient in altering school environments and providing health promotion activities. Successful change is largely dependent upon the participation of all involved. Without preparation for change, people will muddle through without a clear concept of what the changes are supposed to be and, more important, what their roles are in such changes.

Staff development programs offering training to school personnel serve as a bridge between current practices and changes toward the ideal. New terms, new policies, new procedures, explanations of benefits and how the organization and school day will be altered are all part of staff development for improving school environments. Staff development programs present the opportunity to focus on change and innovation and to help individuals adapt to change.

Time

Time is also an important consideration. Adequate amounts of time will be needed to effect changes in the school environment. While there is always pressure to act immediately, there are matching pressures to plan and implement change through a participative process. Making organizational change work is messy, often seemingly unproductive, and time consuming. Program implementation, activities and evaluation must be given time and allowed to develop to the point where effects can be discerned.

In corporate environments, health promotion programs have been effective in making important health behavior changes within a three- to five-year period. Behavioral change takes time. Premature efforts to determine success have proved to be the downfall of many health promotion programs, resulting in lost opportunities.

Health Promotion Program Development

Step 1. Take inventory of what is already available.
- health services
- facilities and equipment
- staff capabilities and enthusiasm for participation
- employee benefits to support programs
- quality of physical plant
- community interest in health promotion topics and relationships with the school
- parental involvement
- needs, interests and issues

Step 2. Set priorities.
- Gather information and share results.
- Match available resources with priorities.
- Ask for feedback to determine the final order of priority.
- Initiate what is most desired and needed first.
- Focus on the possibilities for immediate and visible success for the highest priority.

Step 3. Set program goals.
- Realistic goals should be based on the work of the school health council and the information gathered and assessed by it.
- Goals should have specific measurable objectives to guide program activities during implementation.

Step 4. Consider possible program activities.
- smoking prevention and cessation
- alcohol and other drug abuse prevention and intervention
- nutrition programs
- physical fitness and exercise
- stress management
- individual health and safety

Step 5. Implement the program.
- Starter activities can announce the implementation of programs (e.g., an opening ceremony with lots of school participation—school health fair, a health week at school with sequential activities to focus attention on health).
- Health-risk appraisals can help potential participants assess their health status and identify important areas for improvement based on baseline measures of height, weight, blood pressure, etc. Nutrition and exercise counseling can be provided.
- Using baseline measures, subsequent targets and measures of individual progress and overall program effects can be established.
- Individual and group goals should be set, tailoring activities to the specific characteristics of participants.
- Periodic reviews and opportunities for feedback from program participants will maintain interest and participation as well as determine alterations necessary to maintain or increase satisfaction. Such feedback allows programs to make gradual adjustments while maintaining focus.
- Program reassessment (evaluation) involves regular, periodic reviews of the program to determine what is needed to meet objectives or which objectives need to be modified.
- Programs are reinvigorated by altering their format, recognizing changes in program participants, and changing objectives as progress toward a healthier climate is made.

Step 6. Evaluate the program.
- Use initial baseline data and data collected at the end of the program to compare changes with measurable objectives for the program.
- Assess impact on individuals (an intermediate step in summative evaluation). Changes in health status take time but people experience personal benefits in a relatively short time—more energy, better outlook, increased enthusiasm, decreased illness, decreased absenteeism, etc.
- Assess the cost effectiveness of programs. The resources used for programs should be weighed against the results of the program to determine how much program benefits cost.
- Use program results and objectives to make improvements in subsequent program offerings (formative evaluation).
- Use program results and objectives to determine whether a program should be retained or dropped (summative evaluation).

> **Action Steps Timeline**
>
> Needs assessment (Step 1)—2 to 4 months
> Planning (Steps 2, 3 and 4)—3 to 5 months
> Program implementation (Step 5)—Begins 5 to 9 months after start.
> Evaluation (Step 6)—At end of each program activity and at least annually.
>
> The cycle for program development should be repeated every two to three years.

Benefits of Schoolsite Health Promotion Programs

First among the many benefits to be expected from a schoolsite health promotion program is improvement in the morale of the staff. Morale is strongly associated with commitment to the goals and objectives of the organization and is reflected in measurable terms such as absenteeism and productivity. Enthusiastic and capable school personnel in turn inspire and empower students to achieve.

Health promotion programs have had demonstrated effects on many behaviors that are deleterious to health, including smoking, sedentary living, overweight and poor nutrition. Such changes reduce health care costs. Health problems are minimized by a more healthful approach to managing the rigors of working in the school. Health promotion programs also emphasize the importance of the individual staff member and his or her contributions to the school.

The costs of altering the school environment will be more than repaid through the direct and indirect benefits achieved. The success of staff health promotion programs will affect students. Healthy teachers and staff produce a climate of optimism and dedication to the goals and objectives of the school. This positive climate helps alter student expectations of their teachers and other school staff. In turn, students rethink and reorient themselves to their education. Promoting the health of school staff benefits individual staff members, schools and students alike. Health and success at school go hand in hand. By improving the conditions for education and the health status of those who participate in the process, everyone at school wins.

Benefits of Health Promotion

Direct Benefits
- lowered health care costs
- improved productivity
- decreased absenteeism
- improved student performance on standardized measures
- greater commitment to educational goals by staff as well as students
- lower staff recruiting costs

Indirect Benefits
- improved morale among staff and students
- improved image of the school
- greater commitment of parents and community to the school
- attraction of high-quality staff to the school
- greater willingness to accept innovation and change

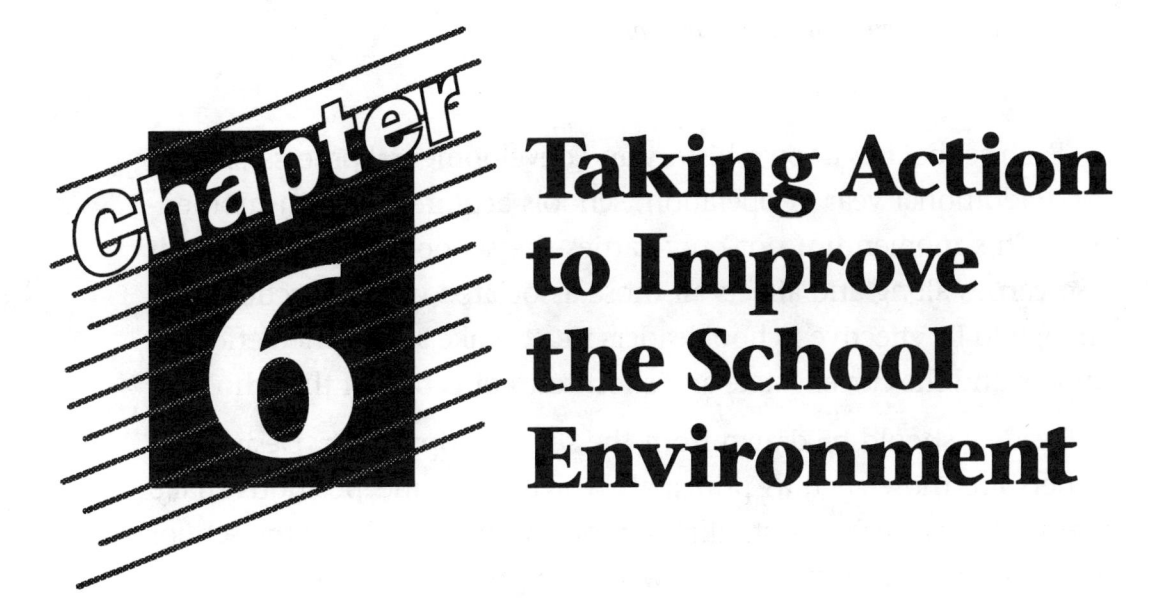

Chapter 6: Taking Action to Improve the School Environment

THE KEY TO IMPROVING the school environment lies in the ability to turn concepts and resources into effective action. Human and material resources must be channeled into a coherent, participative process. The first step in this process involves organizing disparate resources and people for effective action. The next step is to develop a program for promoting health and improving the school environment. The planning, implementation and evaluation stages of a program are all important. In addition to establishing programs and activities to meet stated objectives and goals, school leaders must develop a strategic planning perspective to maintain improvements and respond to changing needs.

Schools *can* take positive steps to improve the total environment of the school. School personnel can be encouraged to make changes to the environment to benefit their students, themselves and others; but school leaders must recognize the need to do so. Steps for improvement begin with the recognition of the value of the students and personnel.

Taking Action to Improve the School Environment

Each school has its own history and developmental processes. With each additional year of operation, schools acquire a certain momentum. This momentum not only carries the school into the future, it also carries along and affects all those associated with the school. For change to be effective, school leaders must make a concerted effort to understand the current state and short-term direction of the school.

Leaders should be drawn from the school population. Designated leaders are those such as principals whose titles and positions make them responsible for substantial portions of the school and the school day. Unofficial leaders are those whose length of service and personal qualities afford them respect and influence beyond their official scope. Unofficial leaders may be school counselors, nurses, health educators or other teachers. Individuals with a historical perspective on the school can offer needed perspective on the direction as well as the possibilities for change. All these leaders must recognize the need to alter and improve the school's physical and social environment.

Forming a School Health Council

The initial focus for change should be the formation of a school health council. School health councils can be comprised of a broad range of interests at the school, including:

- faculty
- administration
- other school staff
- school nurses

- school nutritionists
- school counselors
- students

The council should include representatives of parents or students' other family members. School health councils may also include others from the community with an interest in the health of children and youth. Organizations represented on the school health council might include:

- local health departments
- voluntary health agencies
- health care professionals (e.g., medical or dental society)
- service groups

The Role of the Council

The school health council's task is to obtain an overall view of the health of the school and all within it. This view will allow coordinated efforts to protect and promote health to be planned. School health councils function as information and communication exchange mediums. They enable important events, information exchanges and decisions to occur at the school.

These councils can serve as conduits to pass information from students to faculty and staff and vice versa. They are also in an excellent position to make recommendations for correcting problems or difficulties and improving opportunities for health at school. Councils can provide a source of inspiration, support and reinforcement for healthful changes at the school site, as well as for the personal health practices of faculty, staff and students.

An additional role for the school health council is the essential task of planning, implementing, modifying and evaluating programs to enhance the physical and social climate of the school. This expanded undertaking has not been a traditional role for a school health council. But the need to blend physical and social environmental concerns with activities such as health promotion programs for faculty and staff make it imperative that the school health council use its unique position to help make change possible.

The expanded role of the council does not mean that its basic character will change. It will remain an information-seeking and sharing body within the school. But it will also become involved in the process of planning and implementing specific programs, as well as evaluating programs and results.

The school health council serves as a stable, responsible and responsive force for maintaining perspective and momentum for progress. Councils often form for one specific purpose or need and, after the original reason for organizing has been resolved, later disband or lose relevance. The school health council must be able to organize resources and energy toward a specific goal or objective and then maintain the drive toward attaining all established goals. It must also be ready to revise or alter goals as successful programs progress.

Appointing a Leader

The selection of a leader is a key feature in creating an effective school health council. The leader should occupy a school position that relates to the health needs of students, faculty and staff. Familiarity with health and health-related concerns, as well as a commitment to protecting and improving the health of all at school are essential qualities. The leader should also be familiar with individuals, agencies, organizations and parents from the community who could help the school improve its environment.

The leader acts as a coordinator of the various components affecting health at the school, such as health services, food service, physical education, health instruction and building maintenance. Coordinators have little direct authority, but they have a broad responsibility to obtain information regarding problems and issues and to make recommendations that others with authority can implement.

Without a designated leader, the leadership of the school health council will become diffused among its members. The leader provides a focal point so activities can progress in an orderly manner. Therefore, the leader must be a good communicator and organizer, someone who is able to establish good interpersonal relations with those affected by and those with the power to affect school health programs. The leader will also have to establish procedures for information gathering, analysis and interpretation to help the council do its work.

Such leaders may not be readily identifiable within the school environment. Staff development programs within the school and school district may help to identify a council leader. Alternatively, a consultant familiar with school health issues, and their environmental aspects in particular, could facilitate program development. If a consultant is used, a timeline should be established for conclusion of the outside assistance. A leader from the school should be trained to take over the leadership role when the outside assistance ends.

The most important and immediate task for the designated leader of the school health council is to establish protocols for the planning, implementation and evaluation of school health promotion programs and environmental improvements. Once the foundation factors are in place, it will be possible to proceed with development of specific programs.

Taking Action to Improve the School Environment

> **Creating a Foundation for Change**
>
> **Step 1. Commitment by school administration to provide:**
> - knowledge of what is and vision of what should be
> - support for progress toward goals
> - an atmosphere for learning and achievement
>
> **Step 2. Formation of a school health council with:**
> - membership from the entire school community—students, staff, teachers, administrators, parents, community groups
> - access to information and individuals who can help to identify interests, needs, problems, issues and resources
>
> **Step 3. Selection of a leader with the following characteristics:**
> - commitment to school improvement
> - respect of administrators, staff, teachers and students
> - communication skills
> - ability to foster collaboration among differing interests in and out of school

Planning

One of the most important initial challenges in the planning process is to develop an environment of mutual respect among all parties. The designated council leader is the principal actor in establishing this environment, although the efforts of the leader and the school health council must be supported by the school and district administration.

The leader's deliberate modeling of appropriate behavior can contribute to an improved social climate. Similar modeling by those involved in planning and implementation activities also contributes. School staff often turn to faculty or other staff who are responsible for health aspects for guidance in ways to approach health-related topics and programs.

Planning to improve the school environment requires a systematic method for identifying needs and interests, assessing the current health status of students and staff and the strengths and weaknesses in the current environment, and establishing goals and objectives for health promotion and school improvement programs. In addition, planning requires estimating a time frame for establishing programs and making other needed changes. It also requires estimating the amount of time needed before program effects will be able to be determined. Activities must be carefully matched with the goals and objectives established at the beginning of the planning process. Key resource requirements must be identified, and the current capacity of existing resources must be assessed.

Collecting Data

Part of the information gathering about needs and interests may take the form of either a questionnaire for target audiences to complete or an interview schedule. The interview format will allow more open-ended responses to help identify important considerations.

Data on health status can be derived from physical exams required or completed as part of existing policy. Sick leave use and claims data for school personnel, if available from health insurance carriers, can help offer an overall picture of current concerns and issues. These concerns can be used to determine beginning targets for the program.

Additional information may be acquired through setting aside one or more days for conducting health screenings to determine risk factors (e.g., blood pressure, serum cholesterol, body mass). Health screenings might include a health hazard questionnaire for staff and students. The questionnaire would ask for information about the individual's health history and specific health practices. Outside health professionals and those with an interest in health-related matters affecting children and youth also may be able to provide useful insights and information.

Taking Action to Improve the School Environment

Assessing the Current School Environment

Questionnaires can be developed that ask students and staff to assess the current environment of the school. Topics covered should include:

- the safety of the physical plant, grounds and equipment
- services such as health, counseling and nutrition
- policies and procedures affecting health (e.g., smoking areas on campus)
- other resources
- interest in making the school healthier
- the emotional and social climate of the school

Information gathered from such surveys will help identify and prioritize needs, give insight into student and staff concerns, and suggest which programs or activities will receive the most support.

Setting Goals and Objectives

Once the data are collected, the school health council can begin to set goals and objectives. The process of goal setting should be interactive, involving staff, students and parents. The information collected can be used to identify needs, determine objectives and set priorities.

In addition to starting programs and stating program objectives, goals may be directed toward improving morale and working relationships at the school to help everyone be more productive. Goals should be shaped by the unique circumstances of the school, its location, student and parent population characteristics and resources in the community.

> ## Sample Goals for a School Health Program
>
> - Help staff control weight.
> - Encourage better eating habits for students and staff.
> - Offer staff a smoking-cessation program.
> - Establish a schoolwide drug-free policy that includes tobacco.
> - Improve physical fitness of students and staff.
> - Learn how to better use available health insurance benefits.

Identifying Resources

The school health council will want to identify existing resources that can be used in the program.

Physical resources may include:

- classrooms
- audiovisual equipment
- exercise equipment (e.g., weights, exercise mats)
- lockers and showers
- gymnasium
- swimming pool
- on-site food service preparation area
- cafeteria

Personnel resources may include:

- health educators
- nurses
- physical educators

- nutritionists
- counselors
- benefits personnel
- other human services personnel (e.g., EAP)

In addition, existing programs at the school and in the community can be tapped for health promotion purposes.

Implementation

Many practical factors must be considered in program implementation. First, the target audience for planned programs must see that the programs are needed. For example, if weight-loss or smoking-cessation programs for school staff are considered important, then staff must see the need for their participation. They must also see that their commitment of time and energy will lead to successful outcomes.

Staff will assess the importance of these programs and base their commitment on the kinds of commitment that the school is likely to make in support of them. This often boils down to the question of whose time is to be spent on the program. If the school is willing to make the program available to staff during the school day, then staff are more likely to see that there is an important commitment by the school to encourage these activities.

Second, any change in activities at school will be considered in light of current conditions. Are the changes compatible with the existing pattern of the school day? Are the proposals perceived to be an improvement over existing practices? Will the school's reputation be enhanced by participating in new programs for promoting health at school? Lastly, is this simply a tacked-on scheme or is it part of a systematic change occurring in the school environment that is likely to be sustained over time? Answers to these questions are crucial to the adoption of any proposed program.

The impact of the changes on the total school environment must be considered if a program is to succeed. Implementation may require training and orientation sessions for students, faculty and staff, for example. At these sessions, objectives, purposes and procedures can be discussed and preparations for change can be made.

Providing opportunities for feedback from those involved is another important part of implementation. Despite care taken in planning and the logic of change, target audiences' actual experiences with programs are likely to be other than anticipated. Therefore, successful implementation needs procedures for feedback and communication. Because of the changing nature of student populations and social conditions, a program may exhibit a great deal of variation from conceptualization to execution.

Preparations for implementation and modification of programs are further complicated when community groups and agencies and parents are involved with the changes. Complications can occur when the school schedule does not coincide with the schedules of community organizations offering services. Each agency has its own priorities and demands on its resources. Parents may wish to participate in the process, but many find it difficult to schedule enough time to fully participate. Depending upon the level of involvement, a program with parental participation can take more time than one confined to school personnel who spend their days at the school site.

Recruitment can help by targeting parents and community experts and organizations with specific capabilities who also have the time and commitment for participation. While it is desirable to have broad-based participation, it is often necessary to have those with particular knowledge, skills and commitment facilitate program development and operations.

The amount of interaction between students and teachers must also be considered in implementation. As a rule, wider and more varied

Taking Action to Improve the School Environment

involvement in any program will necessitate more frequent communications among all those affected. It will also require more involved preparation for program implementation. Direct involvement of those affected by the changes in the initial stages makes it more likely that the program will be accepted and adopted.

Initial Activities

Initial activities should focus on items that are of the most interest to those in the school, have the potential for immediate success, and are the most visible. Focusing on visible, popular and more easily accomplished objectives establishes a foundation for success. Many important and difficult changes in the social and physical environment will require time and resources. Activities that offer opportunities for initial success and progress are of more practical importance for program success in the early stages than those activities that ultimately may yield greater health benefits.

Timeliness and visibility of change will help those affected to associate enthusiasm and support for change with actual changes in the environment. Initial visible successes reinforce both the need for change and the commitment to improving the school environment. Time spent on complex, long-range tasks runs the risk of expending commitment and energy on outcomes that seem more remote and less relevant to day-to-day conditions.

Initial activities may be as simple as painting buildings and rooms, changing the cafeteria menu to include more nutritious items or menus, establishing an organized after-school walking program for staff, opening the gymnasium to after-hours activities for campus groups, or changing school policy to prohibit tobacco use on campus. These simple steps indicate that plans are being acted on and that further progress is likely. And while these changes may be only a small part of the ultimate desired outcome of improving the physical, psychological and social climates, they do encourage commitment and support. This support then allows other, more complex programs to be carefully designed and implemented.

> **Suggested Initial Activities**
>
> - Experiment with the daily schedule of the school.
> - Use inservice days for stress management and nutritional counseling for staff.
> - Offer smoking-cessation programs or plan a "smoke-free" campus.
> - Allow staff to use sick leave for "healthy days."
> - Use the campus as a site for a community health fair.
> - Use gym facilities for an aerobics program.
> - Plan walking routes for staff before, during and after school.
> - Begin planning for healthier cafeteria menus.

Correcting Physical Hazards

In any program to improve a school's physical environment, first consideration should be given to identifying and correcting physical hazards. The life cycle of many parts of school buildings can be estimated and budgeted for replacement. However, in recent years, the infrastructures of schools have often taken a back seat to other demands, such as new instructional programs to meet compelling educational needs.

At some point, if unattended to, the physical plant's hazards to its occupants may result in unavoidable and unfortunate personal or property damage requiring immediate correction. Many health and safety hazards are often silent until changing circumstances reveal them. As the school environment is altered or compromised, these threats may become evident.

Taking Action to Improve the School Environment

Decisive action toward correcting physical hazards demonstrates the school's commitment to the health and welfare of its students and staff. Such efforts go a long way toward generating support for change and make it easier to implement programs to improve the social environment.

Physical Hazards in the Schools

- worn or dangerous building materials (e.g., uneven gym floors or non-fireretardant draperies)
- broken or inadequate ventilation systems
- holes in playing fields
- broken toilets
- leaking faucets and water coolers
- asbestos ceiling or floor tiles
- rickety stair railings and slippery, worn steps
- inoperable communications systems
- poorly maintained fire hoses and fire extinguishers

Profiting from the Experiences of Others

The experiences of other schools and school districts can be a valuable source of information. As healthy school environments are created and modified, accumulated experiences will provide rich resources for use in planning, implementation and assessment at other schools. Examining programs and strategies that succeed or fail helps others learn what works and adapt strategies and programs to conserve scarce resources.

Given the time and resource constraints that are so much a part of contemporary education, the adoption or adaptation of existing programs to improve school environment may be the most useful means for change. A lack of institutional experience may make it difficult for school leaders to design new initiatives; and identifying and working through problems and issues requires time and energy.

The same amount of effort can be used to seek out existing programs and individuals in other schools or community agencies with experience in improving physical and social environments or establishing health promotion programs. When taking advantage of the experiences of others, the challenge is to adapt programs from other venues to the needs and interests of the specific school in question.

Numerous commercial vendors offer health promotion programs. Many corporate environments have implemented health promotion programs to improve employee health status through organized behavioral change programs. These endeavors include stress management, weight control, exercise, and smoking cessation. They sometimes are linked to employee assistance programs for those with alcohol or drug problems.

Some programs, such as Johnson and Johnson's Stay Well, have used employee health experiences to evaluate the effectiveness of such programs. Stay Well is a comprehensive health promotion program initiated several years ago by the Johnson and Johnson Company. The program is well designed and uses recommended procedures to assess needs, carefully plan programs within the context of the corporate environment, and implement these programs in a way that maximizes employee participation during the working day.

In addition to the planned program activities and the careful collection of data from program participants, it is important to note the company's corporate perspective on the value of its employees. The company views its employees as vital to the success of the corporation and believes that these vital assets should be protected and developed as much as or more than any of the technologies employed in conducting the company's business. Stay Well demonstrated that well-

Taking Action to Improve the School Environment

designed and well-implemented programs result in reduced absenteeism, lower employee turnover, fewer sick days and less use of health care services. These changes lead to savings greater than merely recovering the cost of the program.

Schools may also look to school staff with expertise in one or more areas for help in developing health promotion programs. Schools are particularly well suited for health promotion activities. They have appropriate facilities, such as classrooms, gymnasia and cafeterias. Moreover, schools typically have personnel with training in many areas who can help to design a custom program for the particular needs of the school population. These personnel include:

- health educators
- physical educators
- nurses
- dietitians
- guidance counselors

The expertise of these personnel can enable a school to develop a comprehensive program with a minimal amount of outside labor.

Evaluation

Once programs have been accepted and implemented, their success should be evaluated. Evaluating a program means comparing the results of implementation with the objectives established for the program.

Changing school environment involves numerous objectives. It may mean altering the physical environment—for example, improving available equipment. Success in this area can be determined through a relatively mechanistic process. Similarly, health promotion program successes can be measured by such factors as turnover and absenteeism rates. However, a three-to five-year process is necessary before evidence of these changes can be expected. Other indicators may be changes in school lunch menus or the availability of after-school activities such as exercise and stress-reduction programs for students and staff. Finally, less definite but equally important, data from program participants and measures of satisfaction among all school personnel and students can be obtained.

While objectives and measures are important to the evaluation process, the overall purpose of evaluation must be determined during program planning. There are basically two forms of evaluation: formative and summative.

Formative evaluation is concerned with program improvement. Attention is paid to how the program was implemented, how results of the program deviated from objectives, and how the program was received. Formative evaluation looks at how a program was conducted and what outcomes can be determined. It looks at improving what is being done. Items looked at include the level of satisfaction of program participants, how the program fit into existing schedules and the ways in which the program was conducted.

In contrast, summative evaluation examines the success of the program in meeting objectives, with an interest in proving the merit or worth of the program. Summative evaluation looks at how much of a difference a program has made. Did people quit smoking? Did the number of sick days used decline? Did people lose weight or lower blood pressure or cholesterol levels? Summative evaluation attempts to determine whether or not a program made a difference and whether it should be retained.

It may be possible for both forms of evaluation to be used in assessing programs to improve school environments, but it should be remembered that they are quite different. The purposes of evaluation should be specified as part of the planning process.

Taking Action to Improve the School Environment

Evaluation will make it possible for programs to improve over time as well. Evaluation allows one priority to be substituted for another as conditions or priorities change. Without some form of systematic assessment that can produce measurable evidence of effects, enthusiasm and support for programs may wane.

Responding to Change

In the past few years, schools have experienced dramatic changes affecting students, faculty, staff and administrators alike:

- Average class sizes have increased.
- School budgets have failed to keep pace with either enrollment growth or costs of education.
- Pressure for reducing teacher salaries has increased due to budgetary problems.
- National efforts to standardize the teaching profession have begun.
- Demographics of school-age children and youth have changed.
- Employee benefits have been reduced through "cafeteria" plans, largely driven by increasing medical insurance costs.
- New initiatives for school choice have been proposed and placed on state election ballots.

Building new schools serves and involves many individual and community interests, including school board members, architects, administrators, community leaders from government and business, and parents and parent organizations. Each group helps to shape the location of schools, the physical features of the buildings, and the parts of the community from which students are drawn.

Once built, however, schools are not readily movable. Over the years, communities change, and demand for classroom space increases and decreases. These variations in size may mean some schools burst with students while other schools in the same district have shrinking numbers. Solutions to such problems are not always easy to agree upon.

Students' backgrounds also change. Schools often find that demographic profiles have changed over the years. The numbers of students from various economic, social, cultural and ethnic backgrounds increase or decrease according to national population trends. For example, multicultural school populations, speaking languages other than English, have changed the demographic characteristics of many of our nation's schools and school districts.

Seventy-five percent of the nation's population is urbanized, and much attention has been given to the conditions of education in urban areas. But schools and school districts are now trying to keep up with the process of suburbanization and exurbanization as new towns and cities locate near but apart from traditional urban areas. The needs of inner-city schools have increased as scarce educational resources have been allocated to meet the demands of new populations in new locations.

Rural areas, with their relatively sparse populations scattered over large geographic areas, have their own special needs. As the character of urban/suburban areas has changed, so has rural America. Demographic changes in rural populations have made it difficult for many areas to sustain local schools and to maintain the traditional, important community role of the school in rural areas.

Such changes have a significant impact on school curricula. Changes in curricula can be even more controversial than changes in the configuration of the school and the school day. These changes are often combined with demands to solve the need for physical space. As a consequence, some schools must adapt in almost all their aspects to be able to fulfill their responsibility for educating youth.

Changes in law and in educational philosophy have demanded and encouraged the mainstreaming of students with disabilities into the schools. Equal employment opportunity statutes have also made it possible for those with physical disabilities to acquire teaching and administrative credentials to work in schools. School facilities have had to be modified or designed to accommodate these changes. These social shifts have necessitated changes in the scheduling of the school day and changes in transportation to accommodate students and personnel with mobility limitations. These changes also demand vigilance in maintaining school buildings, grounds and equipment where hazards that would affect those with some form of disability could arise.

The issues and challenges facing education in our country continue to evolve, as do the social conditions for families and communities. In this climate of change, it is unwise to continue to attempt to do business as usual in any field, including health promotion initiatives and other improvements to school environment. Organizations such as schools are challenged to change as society continues to evolve. Institutions that fail to adapt to changing conditions decline. School leaders need to be able to adapt their organizations to the changing nature of education, students, personnel and the communities served by the school. They also need to recognize that changing the way things are done has a significant impact on the school.

To prepare for inevitable change, a process of continual planning, implementation and evaluation must be incorporated into the daily activities of the school. This process must involve all members of the school community—faculty, staff, students, administrators, parents and community organizations, and it must become part of the organization of the school itself. Health promotion and school improvement programs that are simply tacked on to the school routine will be viewed as temporary, worthwhile and timely though they may be. Similarly, if environmental improvement is dependent upon external sources of funds for resources and personnel, then it is also quite likely that these programs will be viewed as temporary. Environmental improvements must become part of the core activities and values of the school. This process takes conscious effort by all those interested in the health of those at school—most important, by the official leadership of the school.

Strategic Planning

A strategic perspective is essential to meet the challenges of change and social evolution in and out of school. A strategic plan ensures that an organization is evolving in the agreed-upon direction. But a successful strategic plan requires a process for creating the plan *and* a process for using it. The strategic plan should be a useful, working document.

Strategic plans are most useful if they are reviewed annually. During this review, activities can be assessed to see if they have led to achieving stated objectives. The continuing relevance of goals and objectives and any need for revision can also be assessed. Revision of goals and objectives will result in changes to activities. Ideally, an annual review enables school leaders to continue the process of improving the school environment while addressing the changing needs of students, parents, staff, teachers, administrators and the surrounding community.

There are many forms of strategic planning. Appendix C presents an outline for a strategic plan that can be used both for initial planning and for subsequent revisions as programs and events progress. An annual review of each component, with particular attention paid to activities, is a key feature of such a plan. Components and timelines should change as situations change.

Special Considerations

As complex, ambitious and time consuming as developing health promotion programs is, there are further considerations necessary if change processes are to achieve their intended effects. Schools are found in every locale—urban, suburban, and rural—within homogeneous as well as heterogeneous communities. Some schools reflect the characteristics of their communities in students, staff, faculty and administrators. Other schools are more diverse, and students, faculty, staff and administrators do not share a common background.

School locations can be remote or in the neighborhood. Schools can be located in supportive, indifferent or hostile communities. Communities may have sparse, rural, homogeneous or dense, urban, heterogeneous populations. All of these factors must be taken into account if any strategic changes in the school are to be successful.

Strategies for developing health promotion programs and for improving school climate are applicable regardless of the settings. Procedures for assessing needs, planning programs, implementing and evaluating them do not have to be changed, either. What is needed, however, is sensitivity to the particular situation of the specific school. Outcomes of environmental improvements will be different depending on the characteristics of the school and community. Priorities within each school environment will be different. Local situations will enable some schools to move faster than others.

Procedures for change and program development must respect cultural, ethnic, socioeconomic and other similarities and differences among those at the school. Where there are significant differences between the backgrounds of school personnel and students, differences must be acknowledged and incorporated into the processes of program development.

Other considerations include the logistics of the school day. How long does it take to get to and from school daily? How do you make environmental changes that need parental involvement when students are bused across town and not enrolled in a neighborhood school? What staff development programs are needed if community demographics change while teachers and administrators remain the same? What happens to programs when there is frequent faculty and staff turnover? If the school is located in a hostile environment, how relevant are health promotion programs to students, faculty, staff and administrators, as well as parents and community members, when basic safety needs are scarcely met? In areas with economic problems, how can the community support its schools?

The characteristics of the school and where it is located cannot be ignored as part of the program planning process. Many urban, inner-city schools are configured as fortresses in an apparent attempt to provide a safe environment for learning. These safety precautions create a fortress atmosphere rather than the teaching/learning environment that is the textbook vision for education. To improve the school climate in such a venue is a formidable task for school personnel, parents, students and community members alike; but it *is* possible. Cooperation among all the main actors is necessary to overcome physical, mental and social barriers when schools are located in hostile community environments.

The next chapter looks at how various schools have answered or at least addressed these questions. In viewing schools to see what they have been doing, we will also see things that should not be done, actions that are deleterious to the well-being of the school as a whole and to its students, faculty and staff. Examples of useful strategies and plans give us guideposts for making improvements.

We must always remember, however, that school environments are dynamic and always in a process of change. School experiences of the past are not the same as today's. And, for better or for worse, today's environments will certainly not be the same as tomorrow's. Nevertheless, it is the underlying thesis of this book that improvements can be made in the dynamic school environment when there is conscious and conscientious recognition of the need for planning and implementing the changes.

Chapter 7
Success Stories: Making Things Work

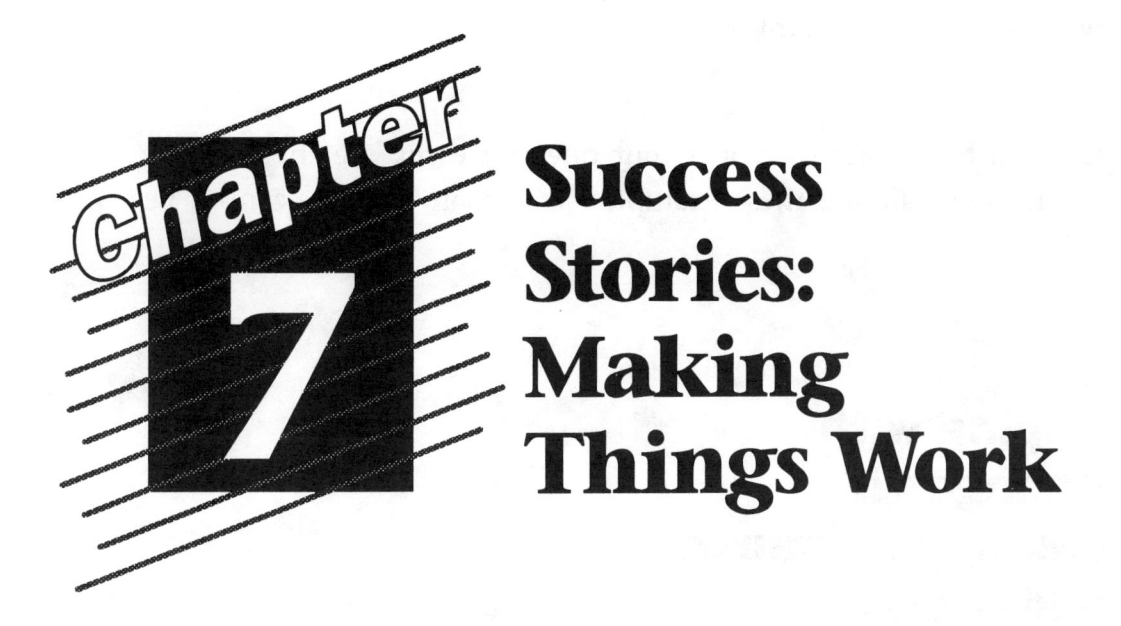

THE PRECEDING CHAPTERS OUTLINE the essential ingredients for improving school environment in broad, general terms. This chapter illustrates the application of these principles within the context of current conditions of education. Many things affect schools today, including changing family structures, demographic features of student populations, violence on and around campuses, student and staff morale, outreach to communities and campus safety. How schools respond to these issues has an important effect on the school environment and, in turn, on student achievement.

The following examples were derived from interactions with teachers and other school personnel over a period of years. They represent some of the means school personnel have found to cope and adapt to changing social and school environments. Examples of practices *not* recommended are also included. These examples illustrate the problems certain actions can create for schools. They are provided to help administrators avoid similar pitfalls. The examples that follow are

Success Stories: Making Things Work

sorted into specific categories, but one can easily see the intrinsic relationships among these examples, which, in practice, cannot be separated.

Coping with Changes in Family Structures and Student Populations

American family structures have changed over the years. The nuclear family with two parents, two children and the father as the sole economic provider, the picture that once characterized industrial society, now represents approximately 6 percent of American families.

Role Models Provide Missing Structure

One suburban district has a great many problems associated with lack of family structure and a high degree of transiency among its student population. One third of the students in the high school are housed in foster homes. Administrators and teachers recognized the substantial lack of role models for these students. As a consequence, the school has developed a summer program for incoming ninth graders to build self-esteem and prepare them for high school.

The school goes further by assigning mentor teachers to work with at-risk students. The mentors help students avoid problems by teaching them refusal skills. The school has also developed a health academy, funded by the state, for students interested in health careers linked to community health agencies. Within the health academy,

English and social studies are integrated to make sure students have a comprehensive curriculum in addition to the science and math classes taught in support of the health curriculum.

Rural Growth Brings Many Changes

In another example, in a well-established, formerly rural district, new residential growth and an influx of new population has decidedly changed the school environment. For many years, the students, teachers and administrators came from the same community and had essentially similar backgrounds. In recent years, however, the diversity and numbers of new students have grown dramatically. The community has changed its rural nature and has become a bedroom suburb offering lower-priced housing for commuting workers. In response, the district has had to hire a large number of teachers in a short period of time and open several new schools. These changes have occurred in an increasingly constrained fiscal environment. The district has hired new teachers from out of state who do not share the same background as the students or the established teachers and administrators.

This district has adopted a training strategy for teachers to address the effects of this rapid change. Yet, because the schools have their roots in a traditionally rural and close community, there is resistance to change on the part of established school personnel. New teachers do not live in the community; and, because of their inexperience in teaching and their newness to the state and district, they have few expectations about the district. It is uncertain how the district's training strategy will help school personnel address the differences in their ranks as well as adapt to the changes in the student population.

District personnel have noticed that changes in the student population have produced some tensions among ethnic and racial groups within the schools. New students who come from gang-infested areas have dropped their former animosity and joined together to form new gangs, relying upon their common experience of gang participation.

Success Stories: Making Things Work

To help counter this situation, the district has hired a "conflict manager" to help strengthen conflict resolution skills of students and staff. The district also has a "high risk" counselor who helps identify and plan programs for students who are at risk for problems that affect school performance.

While this district has an excellent reputation for its schools and the involvement of parents, it is clear that the changes in the community due to new residential construction have brought about fundamental changes in the characteristics of the student population, both in numbers and ethnic and racial diversity. The steps the district has taken to recognize and adapt to these fundamental alterations have been much slower than the actual changes. As a result, pressures to adapt have increased as the district changes from a stable, relatively homogeneous, well-established and close educational environment to a much larger and more diverse district because of the shifts in the underlying community.

Tracking Demographic Shifts

One early opportunity for districts to adapt to such changes is to keep track of the changing nature of their student populations as students enter school, particularly at the early elementary levels. Another district has tracked changes in the demographic characteristics of its students. Consequently, the district is able to use this information as part of the continuing planning process for programs and replacement of teachers and staff. Another strategy is to use staff training programs as a means for identifying and addressing unmet needs and changes among students and their families.

While this kind of planning allows an orderly means for adapting to change, rapid changes in the community may counter planned efforts. One district recognized that economic and demographic changes were producing an environment ripe for gang activity and related violence. As a countermeasure, the district began an "anti-gang" curriculum program in the second grade that continued into high school. Unfortunately, however, many transient students came into the district who did not benefit from the program. This fact, coupled with changes in the community environment, actually resulted in *increased* gang activity and violence in the area surrounding the high school.

Urban Changes and the Problems with Busing

As a final example, a high school in a very large, urban school district experienced demographic changes that led from diversity to ethnic homogeneity. In fact, the numbers of high school age youth increased so much that students from the community had to be bused to other high schools. Within the high school, homogeneity eliminated many of the problems with relationships between diverse groups that predominated the greater urban area. However, without opportunities to interact with students from different backgrounds, the students in this high school may have difficulty adapting to a more broadly representative area after high school.

Many reasons have been used for justifying the practice of busing. In this example, an increased high school age population exceeded the capacity of the local high school. Because school funding is tight and creating new schools for areas with growing enrollments in large districts where other schools are underutilized is difficult, busing is often proposed as a solution. The solution, however, creates its own set of problems that many school officials may fail to recognize. Bused-in students are treated as outsiders by local students, especially where there are racial, ethnic and economic differences. Busing schedules may make it difficult for these students to participate in clubs, sports and other student activities. Finally, parents of bused youth are not able to participate in school activities. As a result, the environment of the schools may be substantially changed without regard to the needs of the youth or the needs of school personnel who must help bused students to adapt.

Success Stories: Making Things Work

The changing nature of the family, its structure, and its economics, coupled with population changes, has had dramatic effects on the schools and school districts cited; some problems were anticipated and some were not. These examples show that attention must be paid to the changing demographic characteristics of students, families and communities and that program plans must be made and adapted accordingly.

Preventing and Controlling Violence

Within our major urban areas it has become commonplace for random acts of violence to occur near or on school campuses. It is surprising to find that some districts and schools have been slow to develop policies and procedures to control and prevent these events. Even more surprising is the number of schools which treat these events as if they never happened.

Communication Is Essential

In one incident in a large urban high school, neither students nor staff were told that a violent event had occurred even though there were police on campus, SWAT teams arriving and police helicopters circling overhead. This lack of communication produced a great deal of anxiety on the part of teachers and students, as well as a spate of groundless rumors. Teacher attempts to ascertain what happened were rebuffed by the administration. Only by going through a police contact in the city was a teacher able to discover what had happened.

This lack of communication results in students, teachers and staff feeling unable to articulate their concerns and address the signs and symptoms of such unwanted activity. Lack of communication is not confined to violence and weapons; the presence and use of drugs on campus, ethnic and racial tensions, and academic program problems may also be ignored or denied. This pattern of coping with problems reveals an administrative attitude that a quiet campus, no matter how it is achieved, is preferable to one where problems are acknowledged. And yet, problems can only begin to be solved when they are recognized and defined.

Consistency and Impartiality

Policies and procedures work best when they are applied consistently and impartially. At one high school in an urban area, students and staff are well aware that the school's administration approaches acts of violence or possession of weapons on campus according to the reputation of the student(s) involved. If a student is one of the "good" kids (i.e., an able student and/or involved in student activities), he or she will be treated differently than one of the "bad" kids (i.e., an apparent low achiever, outsider or troublemaker).

Students and faculty alike find these differences troubling. The message being sent to students and staff is that these are problems only in context: If the "right" kind of student is involved in this kind of problem, it will be okay—weapons and violence are not such a big deal—but the "wrong" kind of student will be held accountable and deserves to be punished. In such an environment, no wonder many students feel alienated and unvalued by the school. Policies must be consistent and enforced impartially. The behavior should be judged, not the child or youth.

Policies and Programs That Work

Schools that have been successful in controlling and preventing violence and weapons on campus have all adopted explicit codes of conduct that are directly communicated to students. When problems arise, the code is uniformly and objectively applied. Following are some examples of how policies and procedures can work.

On one inner-city campus, administrators and faculty became familiar with the kinds of problems faced in the community by students. They then designed a policy stating that violence or weapons possession would result in immediate suspension from school and a review for possible expulsion. This policy is strictly enforced and the results of its implementation are well known to the students. Student government is included in the process of communicating problems and policies and devising solutions.

The school administration also convenes a parent council to help identify problems that may be able to be addressed at school. In turn, administrators have the opportunity to inform the parent council of what is occurring at the school. Administrators are a visible presence on this campus, readily available to students as well as teachers. This not only facilitates communication, but enables administrators to remain vigilant about the campus and its students and staff.

In another suburban high school district, schools have a written policy regarding weapons, violence and drugs. At the beginning of each school year, an assembly is held to review campus conduct policies. Students and their parents are required to sign a form acknowledging their understanding of the policy. The forms are kept on record. Students are held strictly accountable for their conduct. Incidents of violence or weapon possession result in immediate suspension and referral to the police. Students who are suspended on these grounds must reapply to come back to the same school, while continuing their studies at the district's continuation high school.

Administrators and teachers let students know they have an open door for counseling any student with problems, including drugs. Students may also contact school officials if they feel their friends have problems but won't or can't do anything about them. The school also offers programs in conflict resolution and alcohol and other drug education as part of the regular curriculum. These programs are begun in the surrounding elementary and junior high schools.

In a newly suburbanized district, school district officials and police together developed, with a grant from the state, a "storefront" drop-in counseling center for students. School and police officials acknowledged an increase in juvenile criminal activity as well as other problems that needed to be addressed. The center is staffed by qualified counselors who are experienced in working with youth. In this example, attention was focused away from the school site, and services were designed to help young people discuss their problems and find solutions prior to eruptions of violence. The storefront center is located in a part of the community frequented by many residents; it provides a convenient, open environment for everyone. Because this program is still quite new, statistical results are not yet available, however, students and school personnel all feel positively about the center.

In a well-established farming community, a former football coach recognized that many of his players were having difficulties with relationships and with drugs. He also noticed that the community lacked services designed especially to meet the needs of its youth. He began a program by creating a drop-in center where students could go to spend time away from their troubles and receive peer support and counseling. As the center evolved, students who came for assistance grew and matured as they solved their problems. Many became peer counselors themselves. The center has been self-sustaining for many years and has aided many students at crucial times in their lives.

In all of these cases, the schools recognize that their policies and procedures do not entirely address or eliminate problems of weapons, violence and drugs. These problems continue to exist in the communi-

Success Stories: Making Things Work

ties where their students live. However, student achievement has been on the rise since the development of these policies and programs. Students have come to view their schools as safe havens enabling them to more fully participate in the learning process.

Improving School Safety

As discussed earlier, once built, school facilities are difficult and expensive to change. Yet as students and communities change, physical plants must adapt if they are to meet the challenges of educating children and youth.

An Unobtrusive Barrier

In a suburban area experiencing more-frequent random violence, high school administrators and architects plan to improve physical security by erecting a physical barrier to separate the school site from the surrounding community. Whereas many schools have built chain link fences in reaction to safety concerns, this school is taking pains to ensure that the physical barrier is as unobtrusive as possible, blending with the architecture of the school while still providing maximum safety. School staff and students have participated in the design process. This has, of course, required more time and effort than erecting a fence; but the result will be the retention of an attractive and supportive physical environment for students and staff.

Getting Rid of Graffiti

Graffiti is a common problem plaguing inner-city and suburban areas. Arguments about the merits of graffiti as "art" notwithstanding, the net effect of graffiti is deleterious to the atmosphere of the community and the school. Schools that have an aggressive graffiti abatement policy repeatedly have been perceived as more supportive and less threatening. Schools spend upwards of a $1 million per year in staff time and paint to eradicate graffiti. For some schools, the problem persists, as new "taggers" attempt to perfect their craft. But others become discouraged by the immediate erasure of their work and move on to less-hostile sites. Teachers and administrators report that immediate graffiti eradication enhances the quality of life at their schools.

Planning for Renovation

Many states have programs with separate funding for extensively renovating school facilities. These programs may be particularly useful for older buildings. Many older school buildings have asbestos in ceiling and floor tiles. Government grants can be obtained for removing and replacing asbestos with nonhazardous materials.

During renovation, careful planning and scheduling are important to minimize disruption to school schedules. In one large high school, renovation of the building containing the school library made its holdings unavailable for six months. At another school, the difference between funds allocated for "renovation" versus "new construction" was discovered when it came time to equip the renovated structure. Renovation grants do not provide such funding while those for new construction do.

With careful planning and investigation of funding sources, the net result of renovation is to improve not only the physical school buildings but the social environment as well, as such changes strengthen an atmosphere of support and opportunity.

Success Stories: Making Things Work

Retaining Students

Schools have used numerous strategies for improving retention rates. No single step will automatically improve retention, but each of the following suggestions takes a positive step toward reducing drop-out rates and improving school achievement:

- Promote early recognition of specific educational needs (e.g., Head Start).

- Establish programs for new high school students to help them adapt to the high school experience.

- Provide counseling centers on and off campus. Peer counselors can supplement professional staff.

- Offer training and allow time for "at-risk" mentor teachers to help students who are showing signs of having difficulty with school.

- Schedule curricula into time blocks that allow students to spend more concentrated time on task.

- Involve students of different ethnicities and races in student activities and government to reflect the diversity of the school.

- Acknowledge student achievements.

- Highlight historical and social landmarks for the different races and ethnicities who have contributed to civilization.

- Seek new technologies to provide other avenues to learning, (e.g., pursue a grant for new computer equipment and software).

- Develop magnet schools that emphasize particular curricular or career areas, such as math and science or the performing arts. Popularity of magnet schools often results in competitive admissions within the public schools. Gaining entrance into such a school has been a strong motivating factor for a significant number of students.

Improving Teacher Retention and Morale

In a time of fiscal constraints, retaining teachers and maintaining morale presents a great challenge to school officials. Yet certain schools and districts have been able to achieve both these goals despite a deteriorating economic climate.

Providing Support

When one suburban district had to cut back due to decreases in state support, the initial step was to cut district staff rather than teachers and staff at school sites. Subsequent yearly shortfalls necessitated teacher layoffs. However, because the first cuts were made to district and administrative staff, teachers felt that the district had made fair and appropriate personnel decisions and had attempted to maintain educational opportunities for students and support its teachers.

Another district created support for its schools by scheduling an annual noontime barbecue for all students, parents, teachers and staff. District administrators participate in each event, providing school personnel, students and their families with an opportunity to meet and socialize with district administrators.

Several school districts have adopted health promotion programs that offer many activities, such as physical exercise (walking, aerobics, swimming), smoking cessation, nutrition information and stress reduction for all school staff before, during and after the school day. These districts report fewer absences by staff, lower medical care insurance claims, more productivity and more satisfaction with jobs and the school environment.

Many districts and schools employ the concept of mentor teachers to allow those with particular experience and expertise to educate and

Success Stories: Making Things Work

lead their teaching colleagues. Where these practices have worked best, mentor teachers have been selected based on merit rather than seniority. Where seniority was the determining criterion, the value of the mentor teacher program and the aspiration of other teachers to become mentors were diminished.

Unions: Problems and Advantages

Union policies have an effect on morale and retention of teachers, often outside the purview of schools. For example, a policy of one large urban school district union is to support senior teachers first. When difficulties arise, particularly in economic hard times, newer teachers receive less union support than their more-experienced peers. The situation in this district was further complicated by a substantial reduction in teacher salaries despite an increase in class sizes in the district. The union threatened to strike. With a strike, however, newer, lower-paid teachers would have less capacity to withstand the economic sacrifices and more cause to feel their job security was threatened. These events within the district and union have had a devastating effect on teacher morale and will eventually have an effect on retention of younger teachers.

In another district, however, administrators and the teacher's union work in an atmosphere of mutual respect, created by union leadership's interest in problem solving and by the district's practices of equitable negotiation and decision making. The district involves the union in planning and decision making for fiscal increases as well as decreases. As the district grew rapidly, new teachers were recruited. Now, with economic resources in decline, the district has done its best to retain new staff, sacrificing nonteaching and district personnel before teachers. The district also has attempted to ameliorate its monetary shortfall by applying for grants to support programs and personnel while continuing to meet important student needs.

Working with Community Groups

Many schools have recognized opportunities for preserving and enhancing programs by working with agencies and organizations within their communities. As with activities to retain students, any one of these actions is not sufficient in itself to improve the total school environment, but each small step brings a school closer to meeting its educational goals.

- One suburban high school has developed a health careers program within the school. The program provides curricular opportunities for students interested in health care and links the school to health care providers in the local area who would hire graduates from the high school.

- A rural district established a parent/community reading program where parents and members of community organizations come into the elementary classroom to read to the students on a weekly basis. This program offers parents and community organization members an opportunity to witness what is going on in the school and provide support for their children's education.

- A large urban district has initiated an "adopt-a-school" program that matches district schools with community organizations. The community groups provide important support and assist with instructional programs by providing needed materials and equipment to supplement school resources. The community groups and school officials jointly plan programs and identify needs and areas for improvement in both services and instruction.

- As described earlier, one district has developed a drop-in center for students in the community. The project is jointly sponsored with the police department and supported by a grant. It is designed to prevent and control violence and other related

Success Stories: Making Things Work

problems for young people by providing an open atmosphere, away from parents and school. Joint school and community planning and operation of the center enables officials to better understand the difficulties faced by youth in their community and to adapt school environments and programs to meet their needs and interests.

- In one suburban community, a nonprofit neighborhood health center that offers either low-cost or free health services to whomever comes in has developed linkages with the local schools. Many of the health center's clients are young people who do not want to use their family's physicians or who do not have access to medical care. As part of the health center's activities, staff and trained volunteers visit schools to provide information and educational programs for students. This has enabled the schools to expand their health programs and provide essential information to adolescents.

- In a well-established, stable district, administrators at district and school levels are active participants in community organizations and groups. They routinely participate in service organizations, chambers of commerce, philanthropic groups and voluntary health agencies. Such activities are not only a means of contributing to the community but offer an opportunity to gain the cooperation and assistance of community leaders in support of the schools. Communications and cooperative linkages with community groups help create a supportive environment and an excellent reputation for the schools throughout the community.

Schools form a common core experience for all of us in our society. Much has been done in education to help children and youth achieve more, but much remains to be accomplished. School experiences should be lasting and positive influences for young people throughout their lives, establishing habits of mind that will guide development over a lifespan. These examples illustrate that it is possible for those responsible for our schools—all of us, really—to establish a physically, psychologically and socially supportive environment that facilitates student achievement. Recognition of the vital link between educational attainment and environment is crucial if we are to improve the surroundings that teachers, students, and staff experience each day.

Appendix A: Options for Change

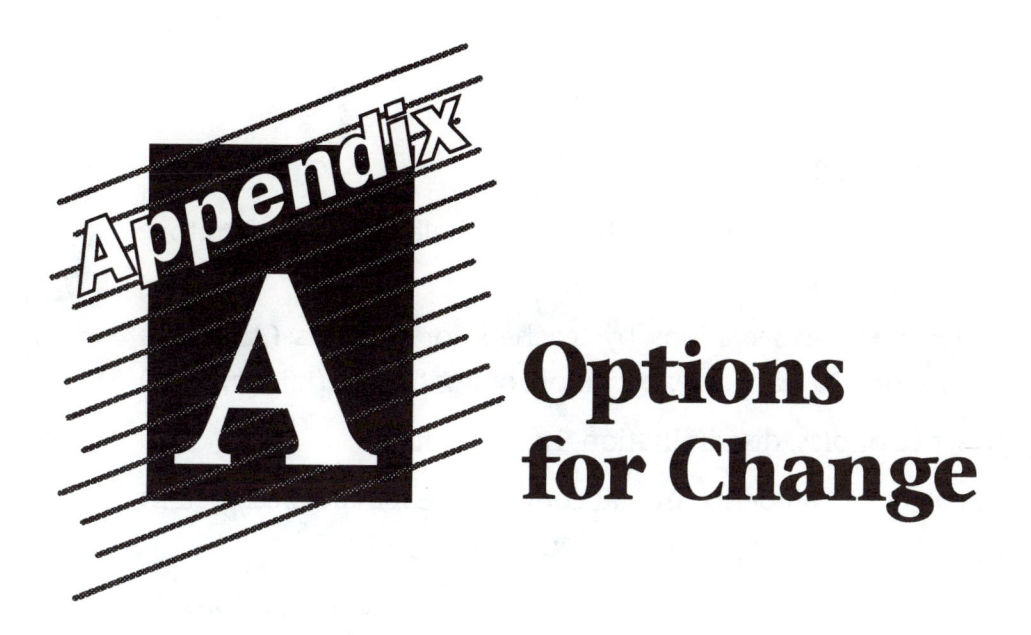

THE FOLLOWING LISTS SUGGEST areas to look at when developing programs to improve the school environment.

Physical Environment

- health and safety (Does the structure meet current codes?)
- condition of the kitchen and cafeteria
- condition of labs, gyms, playgrounds
- overcrowding in classrooms and elsewhere
- physical safety for personnel and students
- tobacco-free and drug-free environment
- condition of equipment, paint and other facility details
- the psychological and social effects of the physical atmosphere

Options for Change

Emotional Climate

- beliefs, values and view of the school held by administrators, teachers, staff and students
- achievement expectations by teachers for students (Are these consistent? Do teachers expect more or less from certain groups?)
- presence of bias, discrimination, homophobia
- acceptance of students into all courses (Are females accepted in auto shop? males in home economics?)
- openness among all at school to the views and opinions of others
- communications (Are these from the bottom up, top down or open?)
- decision making (Do those affected by decisions share in the decision-making process?)
- presence of an "us-versus-them" mentality among students and personnel
- informal leadership (Is this consistent with the goals and objectives established for the school?)
- the degree of inclusion or exclusion of various groups in the daily activities of the school

Social Environment

- policies and procedures (Do these reflect shared beliefs and values of students and staff?)
- recruitment, orientation and retention of new staff
- communication patterns among the primary groups at school and with parents and the community
- modeling by school authorities of responsible, healthy behaviors that are consistent with health instruction

- awards and recognition for contributions that benefit the school and for individual and group achievement
- career development opportunities, continuing education, professional service and sabbatical leave
- opportunities for innovation from parents, students, teachers, staff, administrators

Administrative Concerns

- using the school health council to coordinate activities to ensure consistency
- evaluating progress toward goals and objectives through regular collection of data, information and interviews with school personnel, students, parents and community members
- grants and contracts to support worthwhile projects

Special Considerations

- children at high risk for untreated health problems
- dangerous environments (safety needs)
- health insurance
- reliability of information and sources for health decisions
- links to other aspects of school health program needs, such as pregnancy and parenting, absences due to illness, vision and hearing screening, nutrition and food services

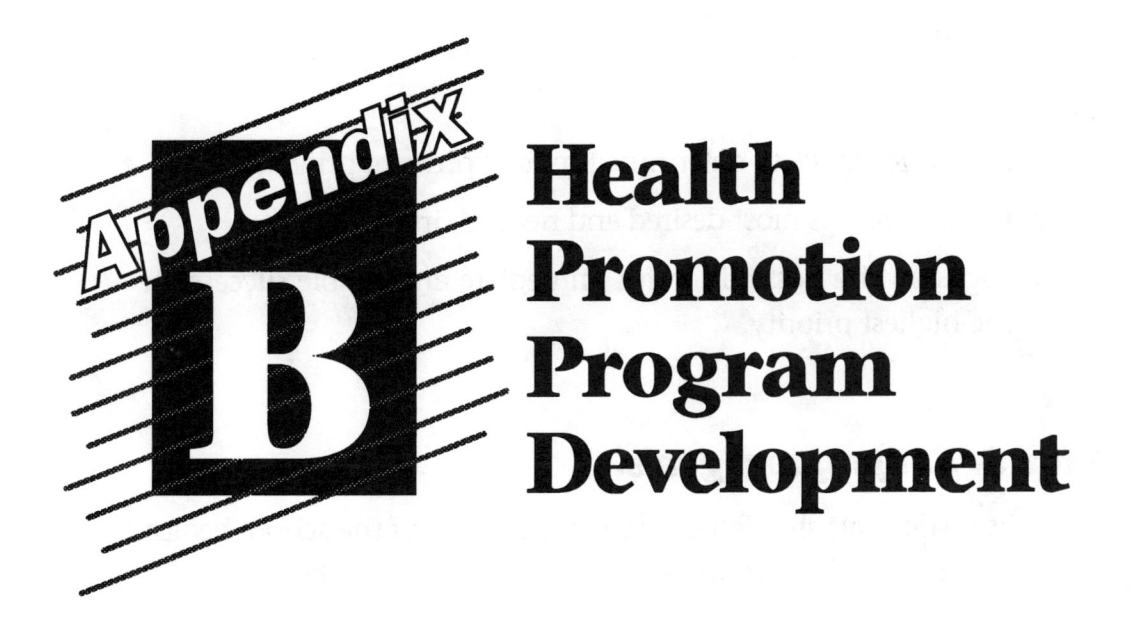

Appendix B: Health Promotion Program Development

Step 1. Take inventory of what is already available.

- health services
- facilities and equipment
- staff capabilities and enthusiasm for participation
- employee benefits to support programs
- quality of physical plant
- community interest in health promotion topics and relationships with the school
- parental involvement
- needs, interests and issues

Step 2. Set priorities.

- Gather information and share results.
- Match available resources with priorities.

Health Promotion Program Development

- Ask for feedback to determine the final order of priority.
- Initiate what is most desired and needed first.
- Focus on the possibilities for immediate and visible success for the highest priority.

Step 3. Set program goals.

- Realistic goals should be based on the work of the school health council and the information gathered and assessed by it.
- Goals should have specific measurable objectives to guide program activities during implementation.

Step 4. Consider possible program activities.

- smoking prevention and cessation
- alcohol and other drug abuse prevention and intervention
- nutrition programs
- physical fitness and exercise
- stress management
- individual health and safety

Step 5. Implement the program.

- Starter activities can announce the implementation of programs (e.g., an opening ceremony with lots of school participation—school health fair, a health week at school with sequential activities to focus attention on health).
- Health-risk appraisals can help potential participants assess their health status and identify important areas for improvement based on baseline measures of height, weight, blood pressure, etc. Nutrition and exercise counseling can be provided.

- Using baseline measures, subsequent targets and measures of individual progress and overall program effects can be established.

- Individual and group goals should be set, tailoring activities to the specific characteristics of participants.

- Periodic reviews and opportunities for feedback from program participants will maintain interest and participation as well as determine alterations necessary to maintain or increase satisfaction. Such feedback allows programs to make gradual adjustments while maintaining focus.

- Program reassessment (evaluation) involves regular, periodic reviews of the program to determine what is needed to meet objectives or which objectives need to be modified.

- Programs are reinvigorated by altering their format, recognizing changes in program participants, and changing objectives as progress toward a healthier climate is made.

Step 6. Evaluate the program.

- Use initial baseline data and data collected at the end of the program to compare changes with measurable objectives for the program.

- Assess impact on individuals (an intermediate step in summative evaluation). Changes in health status take time but people experience personal benefits in a relatively short time—more energy, better outlook, increased enthusiasm, decreased illness, decreased absenteeism, etc.

- Assess the cost effectiveness of programs. The resources used for programs should be weighed against the results of the program to determine how much program benefits cost.

- Use program results and objectives to make improvements in subsequent program offerings (formative evaluation).

- Use program results and objectives to determine whether a program should be retained or dropped (summative evaluation).

Appendix C: Strategic Plan Outline

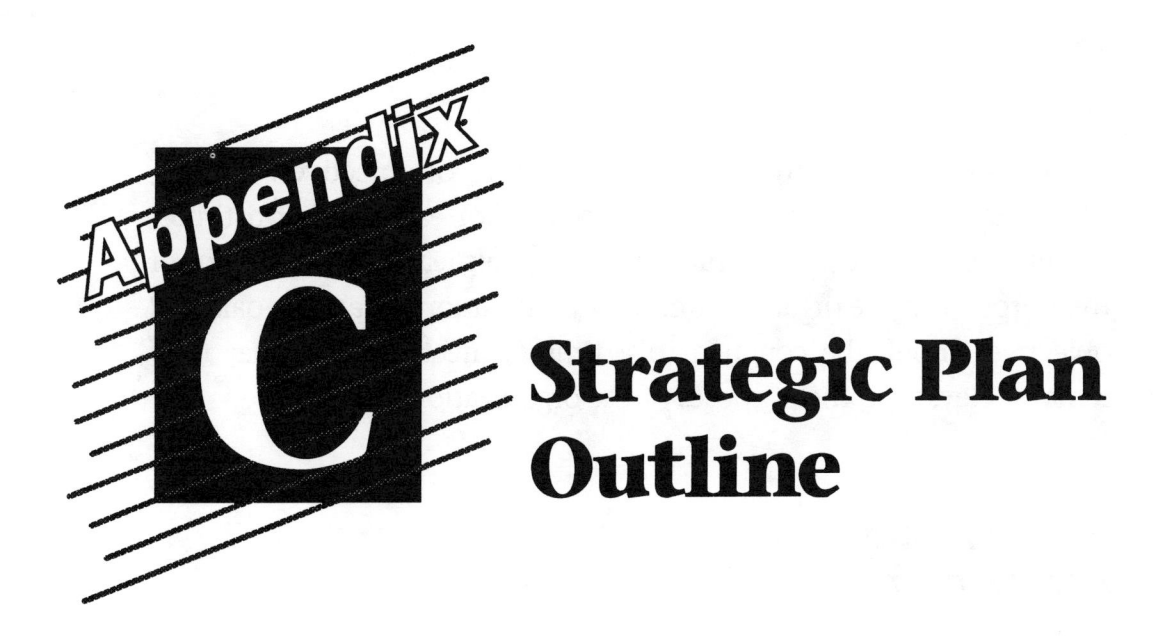

Mission, Goals and Objectives

The mission statement for the school expresses the reasons for its existence and states its purpose. Typically, mission statements are simply stated and direct, but broad in scope. Mission statements rarely change as long as the purposes of the organization remain socially viable. Actions taken to improve school environment should fit within the broad confines of the mission of the school. Relevance to the mission of the organization is essential to programs' continued survival.

Goal statements may be broadly stated, but they must direct organization and activities toward more specific, achievable actions. Goals can change as circumstances and accomplishments dictate. Objectives are specific, achievable steps for organizing and conducting specific activities. Objectives are more temporal than goals. They change as results are achieved or as circumstances change.

Strategic Plan Outline

Specific activities indicate the achievement of objectives. In turn, the achievement of the objectives specified for each goal constitutes achievement of the goal. Achievement of goals leads to attainment of the purposes of the organization. Because situations change, goals and objectives should be couched in a time frame to ensure that they remain relevant to the purposes of the organization.

Environmental Assessment

Any program of improvement must be considered in the context of the current environment of the school and future projections that will affect it. Considerations include:

- school funding
- school voucher proposals
- demographic changes of students
- social responses to particular issues such as HIV/AIDS
- population patterns such as inner-city population declines and increased populations in suburban areas, as well as relocations of populations from one part of the country to another

Changing environmental circumstances affect the ability of the school to offer certain programs and often require the modification of existing programs. They must be taken into account and expressed in specific terms to help guide planning and program development on an ongoing basis.

Strengths and Weaknesses

Every organization has physical, fiscal and human assets as well as deficiencies. Explicit statements identifying pluses and minuses help guide decisions about initiating specific programs and allocating resources for those programs. Programs can attempt to address weaknesses in the school environment or to enhance areas of strength. Identifying strengths and weaknesses explicitly makes it possible to base programs on an appropriate foundation which reflects the realities of the school. As with other components of the strategic plan, strengths and weaknesses will change over time as the school evolves within its social, political and economic context.

Needs and Interests Assessment

Periodic assessment of the interests and needs of those for whom programs are intended is an important component of strategic planning. It is also a means of assessing past program successes. Needs and interests provide information for program planning, in addition to the information obtained from health statistics, medical care insurance and the like.

Staff Training

Educators who are well versed in many aspects of comprehensive school health promotion and environmental improvement programs are a valuable asset. These educators include nurses, dietitians, physical educators, health educators, counselors and others. However, not all schools have these personnel. There are also differences between educating adults and educating children and youth. Explicit identification of staff training needs and programs designed to meet these needs helps maintain program viability and ensures a population of trained adults who can in turn educate and promote the health of students.

Strategic Plan Outline

Activities

Program activities are designed to achieve specific purposes determined by the school health council with input from the school community in its broadest sense. Programs, by their nature, have limits determined by resources, objectives, needs and interests of the audiences, and the timelines needed to achieve their purposes. Each planned activity should have a projected date for accomplishment, and each activity should be assessed at least annually to determine progress toward the stated objective in a timely manner.

Many factors, both within and beyond the control of those responsible, affect the successes of programs. These factors need to be evaluated so that adjustments can be made either to the program or to the timeline. An annual review of activities allows this assessment and adjustment to occur.

Impact and Outcome Evaluations

Periodic evaluation provides essential feedback for continuing program development in two forms. Impact evaluation allows for a more immediate assessment of programs. Impact evaluation measures include the numbers of participants in each program, participants' satisfaction with what has been offered, and objective measures of change wherever possible. Impact evaluation allows school leaders to modify programs according to the experiences of program participants.

Outcome evaluation offers a more long-term focus and examines important individual and cumulative changes. Outcome evaluation measures may include:

- absenteeism rates
- reductions in medical care use and consequent reduction in costs for conducting education
- improvement in student and faculty productivity

- greater safety in and around the school campus
- increased activities of school/community and school/parent partnerships

Such outcomes take longer to achieve. But they have cumulative effects that are very important to overall progress toward the goal of improving school environment.

Measuring the success of both impacts and outcomes allows those involved to see the immediate effects of efforts to improve the school environment while waiting for long-term results to occur. Evaluation results provide data to help assess other aspects of the strategic plan. The data can also be used to ensure that programmatic and overall interests are met and that all who study and work at the school are benefiting from the programs.

Appendix D: Resources

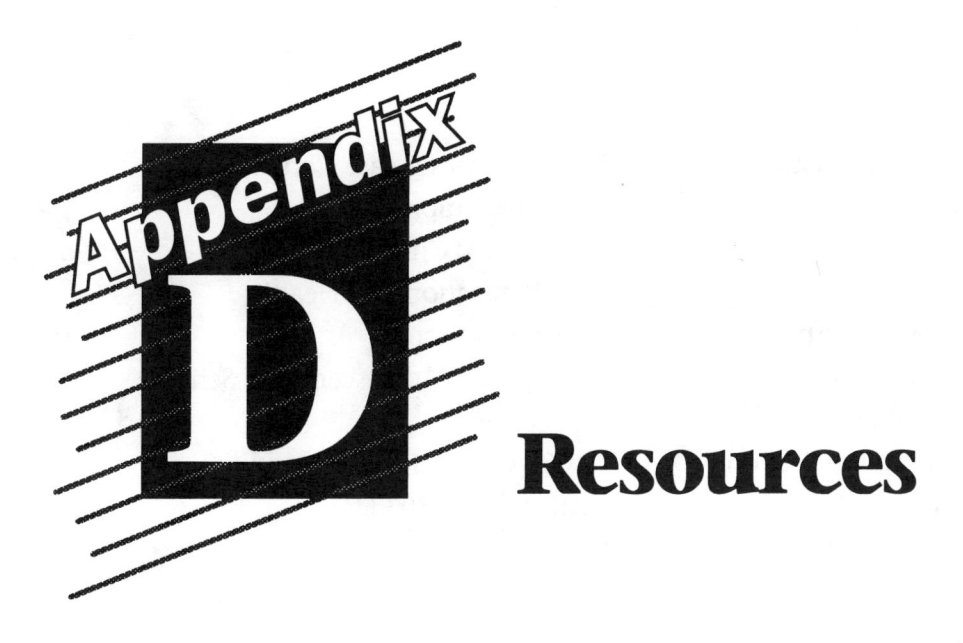

American Academy of Pediatrics
141 Northwest Point Blvd.
Elk Grove, IL 60009

American Cancer Society
3340 Peachtree Rd. NE
Atlanta, GA 30326

American Dental Association
211 East Chicago Ave.
Chicago, IL 60611

American Diabetes Association
2 Park Ave.
New York, NY 10016

American Foundation for AIDS Research (AmFAR)
5900 Wilshire Blvd., 2nd Floor — East Satellite
Los Angeles, CA 90036

American Health Foundation
320 E. 43rd St.
New York, NY 10017

American Heart Association
7320 Greenville Ave.
Dallas, TX 75321

American Institute of Nutrition
9650 Wisconsin Ave.
Washington, DC 20014

Resources

American Lung Association
1740 Broadway
New York, NY 10019

American Public Health
    Association
Public Health Education and
    Health Promotion Section
1015 Fifteenth St. NW
Washington, DC 20005

American School Health
    Association
P.O. Box 708
Kent, OH 44240

Association for the Advancement
    of Health Education
1900 Association Dr.
Reston, VA 22091

Association for Fitness and
    Business
1312 Washington Rd.
Stamford, CT 06902

Asthma and Allergy Foundation of
    America
801 Second Ave.
New York, NY 10017

Centers for Disease Control and
    Prevention
Center for Chronic Disease
    Prevention and Health
    Promotion
Division of Adolescent and School
    Health
1600 Clifton Rd. NE
Atlanta, GA 30333

Clearinghouse for Occupational
    Safety and Health Information
Technical Information Branch
4676 Columbia Parkway
Cincinnati, OH 45226

Consumer Information Center
Pueblo, CO 81009

Food and Drug Administration
Office of Consumer Affairs
5600 Fishers Lane (HFE-88)
Rockville, MD 20857

Juvenile Diabetes Foundation
23 East 26th St.
New York, NY 10017

March of Dimes National
    Foundation
1275 Mamaroneck Ave.
White Plains, NY 10602

Metropolitan Life Insurance
    Company
Health and Safety Division
New York, NY 10010

National AIDS Information
    Clearinghouse
P.O. Box 6003
Rockville, MD 20850

National Cancer Institute
Office of Cancer Communications
Bethesda, MD 20014

National Center for Children in
    Poverty
Columbia University School of
    Public Health
154 Haven Ave.
New York, NY 10032

National Clearinghouse for
    Alcohol and Drug Information
P.O. Box 2345
Rockville, MD 20852

National Council on Alcoholism
12 West 21st St.
New York, NY 10010

National Council on Obesity
P.O. Box 350306
Los Angeles, CA 90035

National Dairy Council
6300 North River Rd.
Rosemont, IL 60018

National Diabetes Information
    Clearinghouse
Box NDIC
Bethesda, MD 20892

National Health Council
622 Third Ave.
New York, NY 10017

National Health Information
    Clearinghouse
P.O. Box 1133
Washington, DC 20013

National High Blood Pressure
    Education Program
Information Center
4733 Bethesda Ave., Room 530
Bethesda, MD 20814

National Mental Health
    Association
1021 Prince St.
Alexandria, VA 22314

National Mental Health Institute
Public Inquiries Branch
5600 Fishers Lane, Room 15C-05
Rockville, MD 20857

Resources

National Safety Council
425 North Michigan Ave.
Chicago, IL 60611

Office of Health Promotion and
 Disease Prevention
Department of Health and Human
 Services
200 Independence Ave. SW
Washington, DC 20201

ODPHP National Health
 Information Center
P.O. Box 1133
Washington, DC 20013-1133

Office on Smoking and Health
Technical Information Center
5600 Fishers Lane
 Park Bldg., Rm. 1-16
Rockville, MD 20857

President's Council on Physical
 Fitness and Sports
450 5th St. NW, Suite 7103
Washington, DC 20001

Society for Nutrition Education
1700 Broadway
Oakland, CA 94612

Bibliography

Ainley, J., J. Foremen and M. Sheret. 1991. High school factors that influence students to remain in school. *Journal of Educational Research* 85 (2): 23-29.

Allensworth, D. D. 1987. Building community support for quality school health programs. *Journal of School Health* 18 (5): 32-38.

Allensworth, D. D., and L. J. Kolbe. 1987. The comprehensive school health program: Exploring an expanded concept. *Journal of School Health* 57 (10): 409-412.

Allensworth, D. D., and W. Patton. 1990. Promoting school health through coalition building. *Eta Sigma Gamma Monograph Series* 7 (2): 1-89.

American Association of School Administrators. 1987. *Why school health?* Washington, DC.

American School Health Association, Association for the Advancement of Health Education and Society for Public Health Education. 1989. *National Adolescent Student Health Survey.* Oakland, CA: Third Party Press.

Ames, E. E., L. A. Trucano, J. C. Wan and M. H. Harris. 1992. *Designing school health curricula.* Dubuque, IA: William C. Brown.

Anspaugh, D. J., and G. O. Ezell. 1990. *Teaching today's health.* 3d ed. Columbus, OH: Merril.

Association for the Advancement of Health Education. 1992. *Strengthening health education for the 1990s.* Reston, VA.

Bibliography

Bandura, A. 1977. *Social learning theory.* Englewood Cliffs, NJ: Prentice-Hall.

Bean, R. 1992. *The four conditions of self-esteem.* Santa Cruz, CA: ETR Associates.

Bender, S. J., and W. D. Sorochan. 1989. *Teaching elementary health science.* 3d ed. Boston: Jones and Bartlett.

Bernstein, L. R., D. Bellorado and W. Bruvold. 1986. Evaluation of a heart health education curriculum for preschoolers, parents, and teachers. *Health Education* June/July:14-17.

Blair, S., L. Tritsch and S. Kutsch. 1987. Worksite health promotion for school faculty and staff. *Journal of School Health* 57 (10): 469-473.

Bradshaw, R. 1991. Stress management for teachers: A practical approach. *The Clearing House* 65:45-47.

California: The state of our children. 1991. *What's happening to our children?* Los Angeles: Children Now.

California: The state of our children. 1992. *Saving the dream.* Los Angeles: Children Now.

Child Health USA '91. 1991. DHHS Publication No. HRS-M-CH 91-1. Washington, DC.

Cleary, M. J. Restructured schools: Challenges and opportunities for school health education. *Journal of School Health* 61 (4): 172-175.

Cornacchia, H. J., L. K. Olsen and C. J. Nickerson. 1988. *Health in elementary schools.* St. Louis, MO: C. V. Mosby.

Council of Chief State School Officers. 1989. *What are the characteristics and components of effective comprehensive school health programs?* Washington, DC.

Creswell, W. H., and I. M. Newman. 1989. *School health practice.* 9th ed. St. Louis, MO: C. V. Mosby.

Davis, J. H. 1983. A study of the high school principal's role in health education. *Journal of School Health* 53 (10): 610-612.

Delgado-Gaitan, C. 1991. Involving parents in the schools: A process of empowerment. *American Journal of Education* 100 (1): 20-46.

Deputat, Z., and M. S. Pavlovich. 1988. School health programs: A comprehensive plan for implementation. *Health Education,* Oberteuffer Symposium on Administrative Aspects of School Health Education, October-November: 47-53.

Dutton, D. B. 1985. Socioeconomic status and children's health. *Medical Care* 23 (2): 142-154.

Everly, G. S., Jr., and R. H. L. Feldman. 1985. *Occupational health promotion: Health behavior in the workplace.* New York: Wiley.

Felner, R. D., and T. Y. Felner. 1989. Primary prevention programs in the educational context: A transactional-ecological framework and analysis. In *Primary Prevention and Promotion in the Schools,* eds. L. A. Bond and B. E. Compas. Beverly Hills, CA: Sage Publications.

Floyd, J. D., and J. D. Lawson. 1992. Look before you leap: Guidelines and caveats for schoolsite health promotion. *Journal of Health Education* 23 (2): 74-84.

Frost, P. J., L. F. Moore, M. R. Louis, C. C. Lundberg and J. Martin. 1985. *Organizational culture.* Beverly Hills, CA: Sage Publications.

Fuchs, V. R. 1983. *How we live: An economic perspective on Americans from birth to death.* Cambridge, MA: Harvard University Press.

Gingiss, P. L. 1992. Enhancing program implementation and maintenance through a multiphase approach to peer-based staff development. *Journal of School Health* 62 (5): 161-166.

Golaszewski, T. J., M. M Milstein, R. D. Duquette and W. M. London. 1984. Organizational and health manifestations of teacher stress: A preliminary report on the Buffalo teacher stress intervention project. *Journal of School Health* 54 (11): 458-463.

Hamburg, D. A. 1991. *The family crucible and healthy child development.* New York: Carnegie Corporation of New York.

Hamilton, P. A. 1982. *Health care consumerism.* St. Louis, MO: C. V. Mosby.

Health Insurance Association of America/American Council of Life Insurance. 1985. *Wellness at the school worksite: A manual.* Washington, DC.

Iverson, D., and L. H. Kolbe. 1983. Evolution of the national disease prevention and health promotion strategy: Establishing a role for the schools. *Journal of School Health* 53 (5): 284-302.

Joki, R. A. 1988. Health education: Program development and implementation. *Health Education,* Oberteuffer Symposium on Administrative Aspects of School Health Education, October-November: 31-33.

Kernaghan, S. G., and B. E. Giloth. 1988. *Tracking the impact of health promotion on organizations: A key to program survival.* Chicago: American Hospital Association.

Kirst, M. 1989. *Conditions of children in California.* Policy Analysis for California Education (PACE). Palo Alto: SRI International.

Kozol, J. 1981. *On being a teacher.* New York: Continuum Publishing.

Lavin, A. T., G. R. Shapiro and K. S. Weill. 1992. Creating an agenda for school-based health promotion: A review of selected reports. *Journal of School Health* 62 (6): 212-228.

Bibliography

Lovato, C. Y., D. D. Allensworth and F. A. Chan. 1989. *School health in America: An assessment of state policies to protect and improve the health of students.* 5th ed. Kent, OH: American School Health Association.

Luty, E. T. L. 1988. Controversial topics in a health education program. *Health Education,* Oberteuffer Symposium on Administrative Aspects of School Health Education, October-November: 39-45.

McCaul, E. J., L. T. James and W. S. Greaves. 1992. Consequences of dropping out of school: Findings from high school and beyond. *Journal of Educational Research* 85 (4): 198-207.

Meyer, A. D. 1982. Adapting to environmental jolts. *Administrative Science Quarterly* 27:515-537.

Milio, N. 1981. *Promoting health through public policy.* Philadelphia: F. W. Davis.

Miller, C. A., A. Fine, S. Adams-Taylor and L. B. Schorr. 1986. *Monitoring children's health: Key indicators.* Washington, DC: American Public Health Association.

Miller, D. F., and S. K. Telljohann. 1992. *Health education in the elementary school.* Dubuque, IA: William C. Brown.

Mitchell, J. T., and D. J. Willover. 1992. Organizational culture in a good high school. *Journal of Educational Administration* 30 (1): 6-16.

Natale, J. A. 1992. Shopping for health benefits. *The American School Board Journal:* 17-23.

National Center for Educational Statistics. 1991. *The condition of education: Elementary and secondary education.* Washington, DC.

National Commission on the Role of the School and the Community in Improving Adolescent Health. 1990. *Code blue: Uniting for healthier youth.* Washington, DC.

Nelson, B. B., Jr. 1988. Principal's commitment: A key to success. *Health Education,* Oberteuffer Symposium on Administrative Aspects of School Health Education, October-November: 34-35.

Nelson, S. 1986. *How healthy is your school? Guidelines for evaluating school health promotion.* New York: National Center for Health Education.

Nettles, S. M. 1991. Community involvement and disadvantaged students: A review. *Review of Educational Research* 61 (3): 379-406.

Newacheck, P. W., and W. R. Taylor. 1992. Childhood chronic illness: Prevalence, severity, and impact. *American Journal of Public Health* 82 (3): 364-371.

Newman, F. M., R. A. Ruter and M. S. Smith. 1989. Organizational factors that affect school sense of efficacy, community and expectations. *Sociology of Education* 62:221-238.

Nickerson, C. J. 1991. Getting in touch with realities of the classroom and community service agencies. *Journal of Health Education* 22 (3): 198-199.

Parkinson, R. S., et al. 1982. *Managing health promotion in the workplace: Guidelines for implementation and evaluation.* Palo Alto, CA: Mayfield Publishing.

Perry, C. L. 1984. Health promotion at school: Expanding the potential for prevention. *School Psychology Review* 13 (2): 15-37.

Perry, C. L., D. M. Murray and G. Griffin. 1990. School-based cardiovascular health promotion: The child and adolescent trial for cardiovascular health (CATCH). *Journal of School Health* 60 (8): 406-413.

Pollock, M. B. 1987. *Planning and implementing health education in schools.* Palo Alto: Mayfield Publishing.

Pollock, M. B., and K. Middleton. 1989. *Elementary school health instruction.* 2d ed. St. Louis, MO: C. V. Mosby.

Pruitt, B. E., D. J. Ballard and L. G. Davis. 1990. The school health promotion profile: Measuring a school's health. *Health Education* 21 (5): 20-24.

Recommendations for school health education. 1981. Denver, CO: Education Commission of the States.

Report of the 1990 Joint Committee on Health Education Terminology. *Journal of Health Education* 22 (2): 97-108.

Report of the Task Force on Education of Young Adolescents. 1989. *Turning points: Preparing American youth for the 21st century.* Washington, DC: Carnegie Council on Adolescent Development.

Rose-Culley, M., J. M. Eddy and B. Cinelli. 1989. A study of school health promotion programs: Implications for planning. *Health Values* 13 (6): 21-30.

Scott, W. R. 1981. *Organizations: Rational, natural and open systems.* Englewood Cliffs, NJ: Prentice-Hall.

Simons-Morton, B. G., G. S. Parcel, T. Baranowski, R. Forthofer and N. M. O'Hara. 1991. Promoting physical activity and healthful diet among children: Results of a school-based intervention study. *American Journal of Public Health* 81 (8): 986-991.

Sloan, R. P., J. C. Gruman and J. P. Allegrante. 1987. *Investing in employee health: A guide to effective health promotion in the workplace.* San Francisco: Jossey-Bass.

Smith, W. M., and R. L. Andrews. 1989. *Instructional leadership: How principals make a difference.* Alexandria, VA: Association for Supervision and Curriculum Development.

Trickett, E. J., and D. Birman. 1989. Taking ecology seriously: A community development approach to individually based preventive interventions in schools. In *Primary prevention and promotion in the schools,* eds. L. A. Bond and B. E. Compas. Beverly Hills, CA: Sage Publications.

U.S. Department of Health and Human Services, Public Health Service. 1990. *Healthy people 2000: National health promotion and disease prevention objectives.* DHHS Publication No. (PHS) 91-50212. Washington, DC.

Weinberg, A. D., N. K. Iammarino, L. Laufman and R. Trost. 1992. Cholesterol screening using the school as a worksite. *Journal of School Health* 62 (2): 45-49.

Wentzel, K. R. Social competence at school: Relation between social responsibility and academic achievement. *Review of Educational Research* 61 (1): 1-24.

Be a Leader in Comprehensive School Health with Other Ground-Breaking Guides from ETR Associates!

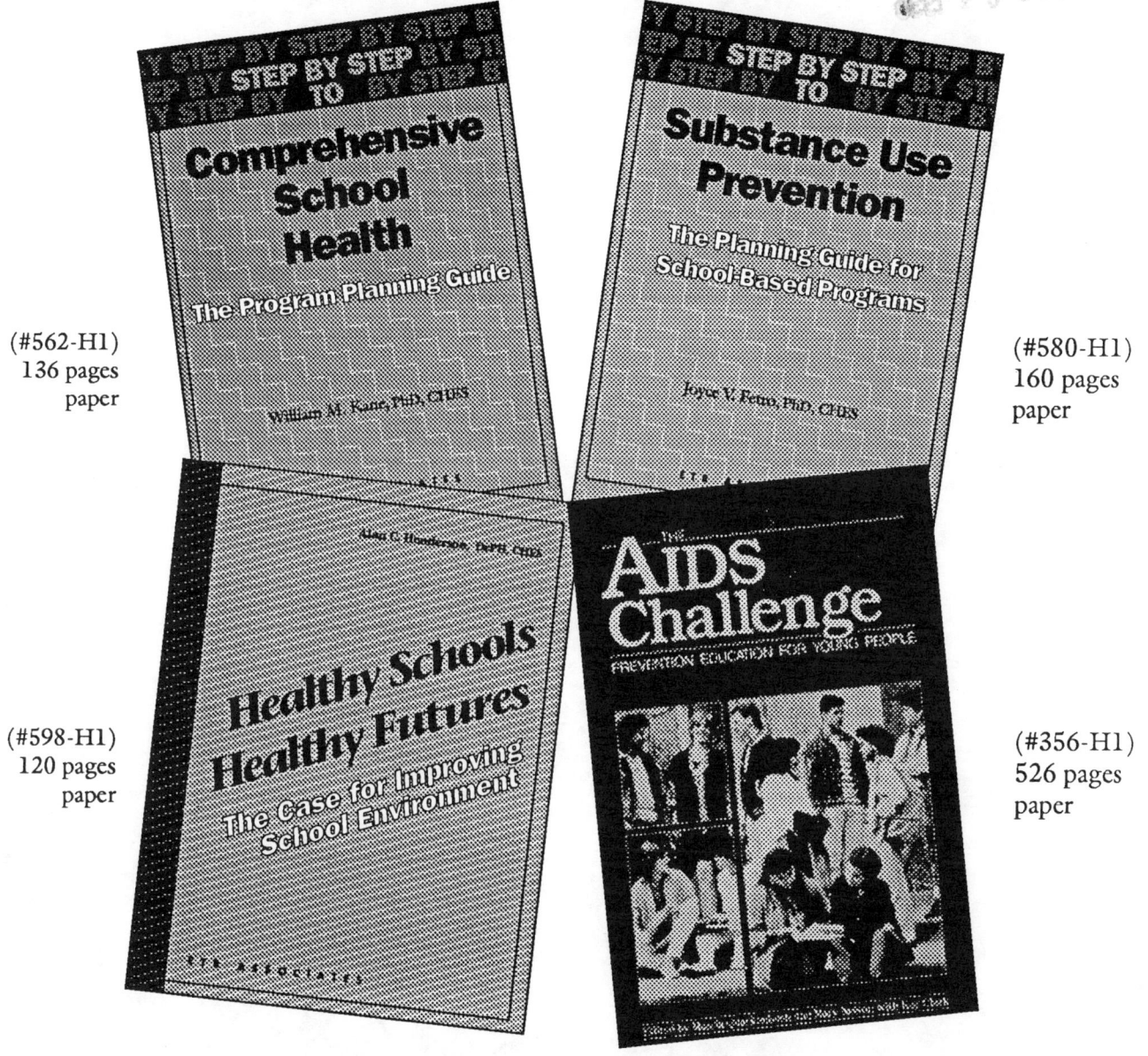

(#562-H1)
136 pages
paper

(#580-H1)
160 pages
paper

(#598-H1)
120 pages
paper

(#356-H1)
526 pages
paper

These are just a few of the more than 600 health education resources available from ETR Associates for today's busy administrators and teachers. Call today for more information on innovative books, curricula, pamphlets and videos!

Call 1 (800) 321-4407

or contact:
Sales Department
ETR Associates, P.O. Box 1830, Santa Cruz, CA 95061-1830

FAX: (408) 438-4284

Prices subject to change without notice.

DEC 04 1996

OCT 1 0 1994
DISCHARGED

DEC 27 1994

OCT 0 9 2008

OCT 0 8 1995

MAY 1995
DISCHARGED

JUL 1996
DISCHARGED

OCT 2 3 1996